INTUITIVE
LIVING

INTUITIVE LIVING

A 6-week guide to self-love, intuitive eating and
reclaiming your mind–body connection

PANDORA PALOMA

S

First published in Great Britain in 2019 by Orion Spring
an imprint of The Orion Publishing Group Ltd
Carmelite House, 50 Victoria Embankment
London EC4Y 0DZ

An Hachette UK Company

1 3 5 7 9 10 8 6 4 2

Every effort has been made to ensure that the information in the book
is accurate. The information in this book may not be applicable in each
individual case so it is advised that professional medical advice is obtained
for specific health matters and before changing any medication or dosage.
Neither the publisher nor author accepts any legal responsibility for any
personal injury or other damage or loss arising from the use of the
information in this book. In addition, if you are concerned about
your diet or exercise regime and wish to change them, you
should consult a health practitioner first.

A CIP catalogue record for this book is
available from the British Library.

ISBN (Trade paperback) 978 1 4091 8441 6
ISBN (eBook) 978 1 4091 8442 3

Printed and bound by CPI Group (UK) Ltd, Croydon, CR0 4YY

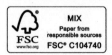

MIX
Paper from
responsible sources
FSC® C104740

www.orionbooks.co.uk

ORION
SPRING

Contents

Foreword

I first met Pandora around five years ago when we were both beginning our new businesses. Back then, no one dared to admit they were 'spiritual', 'intuitive' or even 'meditating'! Oh, how times have changed. Now we're all tree-hugging, crystal-carrying, Palo Santo-burning spiritualistas – it's now cool to be spiritual!

But the thing is, we're ALL spiritual. We ALL have a spirit, a soul and a life force. Just like we have a mind, a body and a heart. So it's great that more and more of us are awakening to this idea and realising it is a big part of who we are.

Life is about remembering who we are and why we're here – a biggie, but when you connect to your spiritual awareness and understanding, you can expand in so many more ways, plus feel more confident, braver and happier than ever. Bonus!

Pandora is a true leader in the (often confusing) world of nutrition. Her down-to-earth and intuitive approach helps you understand yourself on a deep level in the very complex world of food. She is 'rooted' in wisdom and knowledge and oozes insight, which is the best combination and a must-have skill to really understand the human spirit.

To truly comprehend how to 'nourish' yourself, you have to understand the emotional and spiritual aspects of nourishment and the underlying reasons 'why' we do what we do, and 'why' we behave in the way we behave. When you look more closely at this, you'll find we often punish our bodies and, in turn, suppress our spirit or lust for life (our life force).

I heard the term 'spiritually anorexic' a while ago, and it really does sum up the condition of the modern millennial. We are, quite liter-ally, 'starved' spiritually; unable to connect to our bodies and truly *feel* what is happening within them. This means we're unhappy, depressed, anxious and locked in our minds. The way out or way back to a sense of control, and therefore happiness (or so we believe), is frequently to punish ourselves through two of the things we *can* control: food and eating.

Like many of you reading this, I too struggled with an eating disorder in my twenties; trying hard to regain control over my life and wanting to desperately fit in. This is an all too common story and it can only be heightened by the increasing pressure to look amazing on social media and mirror celebrities' lifestyles, for example the Kardashians.

Intuitive Living is the must-buy handbook for increasing your happi-ness in life – physically, emotionally and spiritually. Pandora gives a much-needed medicine to the negative self-talk and chronic disconnec-tion we experience on a daily basis.

What do you love about yourself? By the end of this book, you'll not only know the answer to this question, but you will beam love from every pore and cell of your body. You'll feel so incredible in your mind, body and soul that you'll want to shout it from the rooftops. And that's what we all long for … true fulfilment and epic self-love.

This six-week journey I know, with absolutely certainty, will help so many of you transform not only your lives from the inside out, but the lives of your partners, families and friends too.

When we keep our minds open and stay receptive to new ways of thinking, living, being and interacting with food, we learn more about ourselves, grow into our bodies, expand more than ever, evolve into our purpose and, as Pandora says, 'live a truly remarkable life'.

You're born to inspire. You have a gift. And enjoying a truly intuitive way of living, loving, eating and being is the pathway to true inner inspiration, which will radiate out from you and touch the hearts of every other human you're here to inspire and interact with, including yourself.

So, go on, get 'in-tune', get inspired and go and love your life. Life is for truly living … intuitively, completely and totally.

Be happy, live happy, eat happy.

Welcome to Intuitive Living.

Jody Shield

Introduction

Transform your life to transform your relationship with food, your mind *and* your body.

As a nutritionist and life coach, I've heard a lot of stories about our relationship with food. What I found very early on in my career is that diets don't work. It's never really about the dieting when the focus is finding true health. It's always about the living. I know this myself. From my early teens I was plagued by a desire to be thinner and so I spent much of this time – into my early twenties – trying to make myself smaller, in more ways than just physically. I kept myself small – never wanting to be truly seen or truly heard – people-pleasing to seem 'together'. Food was the behind-the-scenes mechanism for managing this rosy facade; I was together on the outside while controlling, critical and harsh on the inside.

Real health has to start with your life, trusting in your body and mastering your mindset. I trained in traditional nutrition and, while I firmly believe that food can heal, so much of what I felt is what I also see with my clients: women struggling. Yes, with food, but fuelled by how they were living; with limiting beliefs and an overwhelming inner critic. I had been there too. I decided to shift the emphasis of my work to 'living', focusing on transforming how we live and think in order to reshape our relationship with food. When you alter the way you've been living, your relationship with food changes, because you start showing up for your life in a big way.

This book is a response to the common threads that are revealed in the stories of each woman I've worked with – a lack of self-love and compassion, an inner critic that is holding her back, and the lack of trust in herself to listen to her body and her inner guide as the real tool to find true health and satisfaction in life. The movement of Intuitive Living is born and, with this book, I am sharing it with you.

We're living in a time when we're more connected to others than ever before, but I believe we've lost connection with ourselves – and our bodies – as a result. It's time to regain that connection between our mind and our body, so we can learn how to nourish ourselves properly in mind, body and spirit. Intuitive living bridges the gap between mind and body. It reconnects you to areas of your life that you've been hiding from, breaks you free from stories and imprints you've been living and believing and, most importantly, it banishes your toxic self-talk. Your intuition is a guide for life and never before have we needed this so badly. In a world where everyone has an opinion and our views, thoughts and feelings can be shared widely through social media platforms, blogs and Instagram feeds, it can be really hard to see through the noise. It can be difficult to tune in to the thing that really knows what is best for us: intuition. Intuition is the voice that understands, accepts and loves you just as you are.

When it comes to our relationship with eating, food is rarely the centre of the problem. With so much – often contradictory – advice on how we should eat and what it is to be healthy, we've become lost and further from the one thing that really knows these answers to true health: our intuition. From fad diets to hashtag clean eating, we've been living with a ton of rules – eat this, wear that, be like them, work hard, play harder – and it can be really confusing. You know your body and mind better than anyone else. Who are you behind all of these facades? Who are you without all of these rules? It's time to change the narrative, reclaim our mind–body connection and rewrite our story, based on our own journey and guided by our intuition.

This book throws away the diet rulebook and instead introduces the concept that you can become an expert on your own eating and living habits by using your intuition. This concept is one that lasts a lifetime for those hungry for more than just a quick fix. It was learning about nutrition that helped me fix my sh*t around food. I couldn't believe that for so long I had been hating on my body, talking to myself so negatively and denying myself foods that really fed my soul. But I also found that much of the content being brought to me at nutrition school was contradictory in some way. While we learnt a little about the emotional state of the client, I wanted to go deeper. I wanted to know more about their food choices, their mentalities around food and how they affected their life. It was soon after graduating from nutrition school that I trained in Intuitive Living and as a life coach. I wanted to get deep into what made women so afraid of food and their bodies and the ways they were talking to themselves that kept them feeling stuck. Why weren't women celebrating what I believed to be the most incredible vessel, their body?

I've asked many women what they love about themselves. I've seen many women cry at the mere thought of answering. I've waited many minutes for answers. This is why self-love is the basis of my work and this book; because true health starts here. Intuitive eating is inextricably linked to self-love. After all, how we eat and treat ourselves is often indicative of how we're feeling about ourselves. And it's no surprise that with our busy modern lifestyle, taking care of our body is not at the top of the priority list. When you love yourself fully, you direct your attention away from the outside world and back into you. When you engage with self-love and put yourself first, you can bring trusting your intuition into practice.

My clinic has been a playground for discovery. I've tapped into women's stories deeply; the foundations of their limiting beliefs and rules they've quite literally been fed about how they should feel about food and their bodies. I quickly realised I needed to spread my message – the 'living' of health – and I created an online Intuitive Eating and Living Programme, enabling me to hear more stories from around the world and help to re-programme the way women were thinking. I'm proud that as a result of this, women worldwide have experienced positive results including:

- Being more conscious in life
- Trusting in their bodies
- Making food and life choices based on trust, not fear
- Feeling closer to and trusting their inner wisdom: their intuition
- Becoming more aligned to their purpose
- Breaking free from diet mentalities and blocks around their body
- Learning to love themselves, inside and out
- Breaking up with bad habits and limiting beliefs
- Releasing their toxic self-talk and finding a kinder communication with their inner voice
- Finding satisfaction in all areas of life
- Showing up to themselves in their truest form
- To feel, to really feel

The material I teach comes from everything I've learnt in nutrition and life coaching, along with everything I have learnt in life. The tools and techniques are tried and tested by myself and the women I've worked with around the world, devised from the many stories and mentalities I've heard but also from my own complex issues around food and my body. Trust me, you are not alone in how you see your body and how your inner critic fuels much of your decision-making. Taking you through a six-week, step-by-step transformative journey, this book explores self-love, challenging your inner critic, understanding where you've been going wrong in the past, and helping you to understand intuition and the role it plays in eating and living. Are you ready to tap into yours and create your own rules around food, and life?

This book is a journey of self-discovery. With each chapter you'll re-establish a kinder relationship with your body, break free from the ongoing battle with dieting, negative body blocks and mentalities, and feed your soul for a life rich in satisfaction. The chapters are broken down into six or seven sections; the idea being that you read through over a week and allow the content to build your knowledge. Each chapter finishes with tools and techniques for that week, which you can implement throughout the next. By Week 6 you will be well on your way to living intuitively. Some of the tools are very practical, and some might seem a bit 'woo-woo' to you. Give them a chance. I promise I'm on the right side of strange and I've used all of these techniques myself. By engaging with your intuition you can stop faking it and start making it, your way. There's no rulebook to life, and when you start seeing and letting go of everyone else's bullsh*t imprints about body, food and living, you can start creating the life that you want. It's never too late for you to start doing you.

This is the book I wish I'd had in my early twenties. I've written it as a guide for women who want a new perspective on themselves but also on life. It's for yo-yo dieters, people who feel body-shamed, who compare their lives against others on social media, and those who are done with seeing images of people doing yoga poses on a beach that they'll never be able to achieve. It's for those who feel like they've lost their purpose, or their connection to their own body and their intuition. It's for those who want to feel empowered by their body and learn the true meaning of self-love. It's for those who need support with food and those who need nurturing from the inside out. It's for those who want to feel truly satisfied with life.

For this journey together, I simply ask that you open your mind to the possibility that your intuition can guide you so much more than you realise. You can and will – with this book – upgrade your life with the knowledge that is already inside you. If you're serious about exploring and expanding in life, then it's time to trust the voice inside you. It's with this voice that you can create a truly remarkable life. Give your intuition a chance and you'll reward yourself with the biggest gift of your life.

Welcome to Intuitive Living.
Pandora Paloma

Self-love is True Love

Welcome to the Self-love Club
You Are the Centre of Your Universe
Being Healthily Selfish
Love the Skin You're In
Making Space for Love: The Rooted Reset
Self-love: The Toolkit

WELCOME TO THE SELF-LOVE CLUB

The term self-love often gets some eye-rolls and is becoming a bit of a buzzword in the wellness world, but it isn't rocket science; it's our birthright to give back to ourselves each and every day. There is a misconception that self-love is merely a bit of pampering and the occasional yoga class. Sometimes it is, but other times it might be challenging. It might be facing your fears and emotions, surrendering to feelings of vulnerability or stress. It might often feel soothing, but other times it might take work. But in every way, self-love is about meeting your needs and nourishing the person that you are, which helps you to create your intuitive life. The hardest part of self-love is the realisation that it might just be time to start giving back to you. In this chapter we explore self-love as the basis of an intuitive life. When we love ourselves, the feeling flows through our cells, systems and organs on a consistent basis. Living our lives at this level makes us more aware when anyone or anything crosses our path that throws us out of sync. Our intuition responds and when we love ourselves, we sense that response and pay attention to it. There has never been a better time to learn how to live intuitively. We live so outside of ourselves – our minds, our bodies – but they are our greatest guide in life.

So welcome, you've made it to the Self-love Club. You're about to get to know you better than anyone else. The concept of putting yourself first might be completely new to you; you may have dabbled in it but feel like you've temporarily put yourself back down the priority list again, or you may already be a fully fledged member of the club, but need some inspiration to keep going on the love train. Whichever stage you're at, in this chapter I'll be holding your hand like a BFF, showing you why true health and inner wisdom start with loving yourself fully, explaining the power and potential self-love can bring to the rest of your life.

The Intuitive Living principles of self-love are:

- Putting your needs first
- Being happy in your body – the skin you're in
- Looking in the mirror and not seeing every single stretchmark, scar or extra fold of skin as something to be fixed, changed and made smaller
- Embracing the imperfections and knowing it's these that make you unique
- Trusting the timing of your life and being okay with where you are now; your body, your career, your relationship
- Being mindful, loving and gentle with yourself and your body
- Being courageous enough not to hide or be ashamed of how you look
- Keeping yourself at the top of your priority list

WHY SELF-LOVE?

Let's admit it, there are some days when self-love is easier said than done. The fast pace of life gets in the way and there are emails to send, deadlines looming, social and business occasions aplenty, people to meet, places to see, not to mention partners, babies or parents to look after. Not to mention fanny-hair-nail-tan admin. Jeez. Another day goes by and once again you're too busy being everything to everyone else that you've forgotten to be your own BFF. I hear you. Wherever you are, you're part of this club now. This chapter – and this book – is a one-way ticket back to you, a journey to the self, along with a surprise bonus of things you didn't even think you wanted, but that I know you do. It's the foundation of Intuitive Living. Self-love is your new destination for today and every day. It's time for you to do you.

Self-love is the basis of my work because I truly believe that real health starts here; with loving ourselves, our minds and our bodies unconditionally. You can eat all of the right foods, do the right exercise and meditate for hours a day, but if your relationship with yourself isn't based on kindness and compassion, you will never reach true health and you will never thrive in life. Being open to self-love strengthens your intuition and the journey of intuitive living. In order to eat and live intuitively, you must first understand who you are and what your body is telling you. This starts with you getting to know you, so delve into this chapter with an open mind and an open heart for you, and only you.

WHERE DID THE LOVE FOR OURSELVES GO?

Women have come a long way. We can vote, work, go to university, and choose from careers that were formerly reserved for men only – and these things do not come at the expense of a family. Women are making history, challenging men and running the government – a female prime minister, female CEOs, female-only companies, flexitime, better maternity pay; we have come far. However, the male perspective is still prioritised in our culture and much of the media and advertising world is still designed to please men above women. Plus there is the constant scrutiny women are put under and how females are portrayed in the media; how a woman looks often tops her professional or personal successes, or forms the topic of an article that should really be celebrating her achievements.

The daily stream of #fitspo, #goals and #thighgap clutters our feeds and the rise of the 'selfie' continues, adding pressure so that the relationship you have with yourself becomes more and more about how you look and what you wear, rather than who you are inside. Our world can be outwardly focused and full of dead promises. It's a bit like a topical cellulite cream that promises to banish our dimples, but actually just smells a bit like off cheese and costs you a week's worth of food. It's time to get back in the self-love seat and start feeling empowered on your own, without the need for society's permission or approval. It's time to own who you are, guided by your intuition.

From the many clients I've seen in my clinic, I've identified three main roles that women take when it comes to beliefs about their body. From trying to fit into an unattainable ideal of what it is to be beautiful to constantly comparing ourselves against others, we humans are often made to believe that we aren't good enough, smart enough or at all worthy. We never quite feel 'enough'. If this is you, can you start to identify your triggers? What makes you feel not good enough? In letting self-love in throughout this chapter, you are learning to allow yourself to be seen as you truly are. Do any of these resonate with you?

THE BODY BELIEVER

The Body Believer seeks guidance from all the wrong places. This person believes that every advert, marketing campaign and brand has the final say on how we should think and feel about our bodies. Never satisfied with their own body, the Body Believer allows glossy adverts and airbrushed images to convince them that there is something wrong with their body and that it constantly need improving – odours, sizes, shapes, body hair, even the most natural thing like periods. The Body Believer buys the latest products that promise to sculpt and tone, they try each new diet that comes along, and they make time for the latest fitness fad in a bid to obtain the 'perfect' body. On the outside they appear healthy and fit, but on the inside they feel like a duck treading water, paddling ferociously in order to keep up and appear 'perfect'. The constant flux of such unattainable female forms presented by the media has made the Body Believer either afraid of their body or just downright disgusted by it.

THE EXPERT FITTER-INNER

The Expert Fitter-inner lives with the internal battle of judgement; a fierce reality of our modern world. For them, it happens on the street, online, at work, at home and, worst of all, in their own mind. They've spent much of their early years, or for some their whole life, trying to fit in. Wearing a school uniform 'right', being smart enough but not too smart, cool enough but not trying too hard – the battle continues. Then the Expert Fitter-inner gets a career and it starts all over again. They suffer from a split between who they are and who they present to the world in order to fit in and be accepted.

THE COMPARISON JUNKIE

The life of Comparison Junkie is a never-ending cycle. Their life will be perfect when: they look like Gisele, have a house as big as next door, find a husband, get married, get 'that' job, get a promotion, lose two pounds, lose ten pounds, on and on. They compare bodies, material things and lives with anyone who even marginally looks like they are having a better time or living a better life. It may have started as early as childhood. As a baby, perhaps they were compared to their siblings – who's smarter, cuter, more outgoing? Perhaps they were an only child and fully felt the pressure to succeed and shine in all areas; academically, in their extracurricular activities and socially. The Comparison Junkie grew up constantly trying to outdo anyone around them in a bid to be 'better', or attempting to emulate someone else's impressive traits to gain popularity. Comparing ourselves to others is often a by-product of low self-worth and stems from a lack of belief in ourselves and our own unique life path.

You can take it from me, leading the life of a self-proclaimed Expert Fitter-inner is exhausting. This was me for many years, always trying to be the right person for everyone; funny, smart, hard-working, sexy but not too sexy, kind, interesting. This kind of living is soul-sucking and unsustain-able. I was so busy pleasing everyone that I stopped pleasing myself. I didn't listen to my body. I didn't hear what my intuition was trying to tell me.

ACTIVITY: A QUICK COMPARISON CHECK

Keep a journal and write down the last time you compared yourself to someone. Why did you do it? How did it feel? Could this situation have been different? Why did you feel the need to compare yourself? Did jealousy creep in? When you next catch yourself comparing, write down the answers to these questions in your journal.

Comparison can go on forever and it can clog your mind with beliefs that can squash your intuition. Rather than allow the comparison to lead you to despair, take a deep breath and let the comparison go on the exhale – literally imagine it releasing from your body as you exhale. Replace the comparison with compassion and know that you are on the right path and that you are doing your best.

Once you realise that all this body-shaming, judging and comparison is nonsense, you can hone in on your mind and your body. When you live intuitively, you allow yourself to be free and create the life that you want to live. You create the way you want to feel in life. Self-love comes from self-acceptance and the power is in your hands. You may feel like you are being held back by an invisible

---

hand but the truth is, you are often the one who is holding yourself back. If you can't love yourself, how can you love anybody else? If you can't love yourself, how do you expect others to love you? You need to stop looking for validation and acceptance outside of yourself, and realise that it's all within you. You are unique and it's time to tap into your inner wisdom and shine bright.

REDISCOVERING SELF-LOVE

The way we treat ourselves is often a direct reflection of how we feel about ourselves. The way we speak about ourselves says a lot about how much respect we have for who we are. I call that negative voice toxic self-talk or Neggy Nancy (more on that later) and she's a soul-sucker. When you aren't in love with your number one – you – you ignore the body's signals to slow down and take a chill pill. Here's an example of how we ignore loving ourselves in favour of self-sabotage.

You've had a bad day and emotions are running wild. On the way home you stop off and buy some wine and a giant-sized chocolate bar, with a side of ice-cream. Before you've even stepped through the door you've eaten half of the chocolate, and then you slump on the sofa and send yourself into a food and wine coma. Within 30 minutes you feel overfed, tired and woozy, not to mention guilty and ashamed. You head to bed only to wake up sluggish, hungover and feeling just as low as when you left work. If we break this situation down, here's what you've just said to your body:

1. It's not okay to be emotional
2. I'm not going to feel my feelings
3. I'm not going to treat you with respect
4. I don't care about your vitality and health
5. I don't love you

If you were part of the Self-love Club, you might have done something like this. On leaving work you called a friend and talked through the day you'd had while you walked home to let off steam. On arriving, you'd have cooked yourself a nourishing meal, while slowly sipping on a glass of wine. After dinner you'd have run a bath and used that expensive bath oil your mum got you for Christmas, because you knew it was a special occasion and you deserved it. Then, you'd have got yourself an early night, knowing that tomorrow was a new day and that with the kindness you'd given yourself you would no doubt feel better about everything in the morning. If we break this situation down, here's what you've just said to your body:

1. It's OK to be emotional
2. I'm going to allow myself to feel my feelings
3. I'm going to treat you with respect
4. I care about your vitality and health
5. I love you

The magic of self-love is in your hands and it's time for you to take control. Self-love is identifying your own needs and nurturing them. It's feeling your feelings without shame or disregard. Self-love is about being able to assess whether you're ignoring your feelings and emotions, and instead feeding them with food, alcohol or other distractions, rather than facing them head-on. Self-love is rewarding your body and mind with love and care, rather than junk and rejection. Are you ready for more?

YOU ARE THE CENTRE OF YOUR UNIVERSE

The foundation of self-love is knowing that YOU are the centre of your universe. No one else. There is a saying, 'the world does not revolve around you', and I'm here to disprove this notion. Stand up and spin yourself around in a circle. What happened? No matter what direction you turned yourself in, you are still the centre. The rest of the world does react to you. You are the primary source of everything that happens in your life and it's time to step into your true power; your feminine force. Here's why, and how . . .

Your authentic self comes from inside you and no one else. The key to your health and wellbeing comes from inside you, no one else. In Chinese medicine they call it *Qi* and in Ayurveda they call it *Prana*. I call it force and may the force be with YOU. At least 75 per cent of my clients have very similar complaints. They're tired, they don't sleep well, they don't eat as well as they'd like to, they would like to lose that pesky half a stone, they are stressed and they feel like there is not enough time in the day. Many sit in the chair telling me of their nutrition concerns in a confident and professional way, but when asked how they are feeling emotionally, and how they feel about their bodies, they will often burst into tears. At last, someone is seeing them, listening to them and probing them to talk about what's really going on inside. These are women who are trying to have it all and, in the process, they are losing themselves, their *Prana*, their *Qi*, their feminine force. They are living too much in the realms of masculine energy and not enough in the feminine. I ask them to stop trying to be superwoman, and instead become the goddess. Superwoman works to have it all, but the goddess allows time to enjoy life. She lets life come to her.

SOUL GPS HUNT

Being the centre of your universe simply means putting yourself first in order to keep your glass full. It's only when your glass is full that you can be the best version of yourself for everyone else. You can't be your full wonderful self to others if you're running on empty. Learning to love yourself is you giving yourself the commitment, time and space to become and be at the centre of your universe. Are you craving to be back at the top of that priority list? Are you ready to embark on your own soul

GPS hunt? Life becomes so much more inspiring and magical when you do. You'll blossom into your feminine force and really allow it to shine through. You'll become more connected to your intuition and, in turn, feel more in line with your natural flow of life, not the pace of everyone else around you.

Let me pose some questions for you to think about today:

- When was the last time you felt most connected to yourself?
- What does being a woman feel like to you?
- How does it feel to be you in your truest form?

Think about your superpowers here, your true essence and how you feel when you're living in this way. For many of us our set point is stress, self-doubt or self-hatred, or comparing ourselves with others and coming up short. Can you move that point to one of kindness, calmness and self-awareness? It can seem difficult for us to say yes to our pleasure, but pleasure connects us to our soul and our feminine force. This, in turn, guides us to our intuition. From this moment on I want you to be in control of your very own project 'Soul GPS Hunt'. Seek out anything, anyone, any place that makes you feel most connected to yourself, your body and your intuition.

TOOLS TO STEP INTO YOU

With these simple tools, you'll start finding self-love and be on track to feeling more in control, more empowered and more you.

GET IN TOUCH WITH WHO YOU REALLY ARE

In order to be at the centre of your universe, you have to know what it is that you really want. You have to get in touch with yourself and what matters to you. When you know who you are – and what you will and won't stand for – you'll be able to focus on the activities and people that encourage you to respect yourself. Make a list of the things that are important to you and those that aren't. What makes you feel authentic? Once you've identified this, start giving time to those things that make you feel more like you, and less to those that don't.

FORGIVE YOURSELF FOR YOUR MISTAKES

Letting go of the past can be difficult, but in order to respect who you are now and you in your truest form, you must let go of who you may have been before. Acknowledging your responsibility for the mistakes and failures in life should come hand in hand with the willingness to forgive yourself for them. Instead of blaming yourself for the mistakes you committed in the past, try to discover the lessons these failures/ mistakes might have taught you. When finding your intuition, you start to understand the higher purpose underlying each and every one of your failures, as well as knowing what to avoid in order not to make similar mistakes again. The word acceptance can work a lot here. Do whatever you can to forgive yourself for mistakes you've made and say to yourself that you accept them. We've all made mistakes – it's part of life – but those who respect and know themselves fully know how to let those mistakes go. You can never go back; you can only take what's happened and move forward positively. The way I see it you have two choices: let those negative feelings fester in your energy zone, or let them go.

FORGIVE THOSE WHO HAVE HURT YOU

Forgiveness can be tough sometimes, especially if you've been hurt badly. But holding onto that hurt and anger only makes it more difficult to cultivate love within ourselves. Let go of the pain others have caused and you'll open up space in your heart and mind for more positive emotions and experiences. No matter what wrong has been committed against you, forgiving is always better than clinging onto the pain. Write down on a piece of paper the names of those you'd like to forgive and the reasons why. As you write, imagine any pain still stored in the body being completely released and given to the paper. Now burn the paper and watch as the embers fade. The forgiveness has been given.

ALLOW YOURSELF TO BE SEEN

This is probably the most clichéd thing to say but it is 100 per cent true. Don't wait for someone to tell you what to do, what to wear or how to do it, just go and do it. When you start living authentically, everything improves. If you've always wanted to dance like Michael Jackson, sign up to the local dance class. If you've always felt like there's a singer inside you, have a go at karaoke. Want to wear pink? Wear it. Society gives us enough boundaries as it is. Try to tap into your authentic self and radiate that force. To be yourself and allow yourself to be seen in a world that is often trying to mould you into something else is incredibly powerful.

BEING HEALTHILY SELFISH

When I explain to clients that they are the centre of their universe, I'm often greeted with a confused look. It's important to point out here that I'm not asking you to suddenly become selfish and never do anything for anyone else; I'm asking you to create boundaries and become healthily selfish, which is what we'll explore in this section. The ultimate act of self-love is not adding a bunch of things to your schedule but how you organise your schedule. Self-love is knowing and setting your own bound-aries in order to protect your precious time, and your energy. Self-love is learning to say no. Looking after yourself isn't being selfish or a luxury, it's a necessity.

I spent a good chunk of my life saying yes. Yes to work commitments, yes to family parties, yes to friends, men and everything in between. I made time for exercise, and cooking my own food; I launched a business and ran around like a lunatic trying to create the 'perfect' life. I lived in the big city of London where 'having it all' was the mantra of life. I thought

I could be everything I wanted to be and more, and strove hard to get there. I thought that to obtain 'success' meant I had to work hard and play harder. But I was wrong. At this point, I had launched a catering company serving plant-based food to the fashion crews on photoshoots and at events. Delivery could be anytime from 5am to 9am, so I'd often finish late to prep and then be up early to deliver. To fund the business I did other work and I was also teaching yoga three mornings and two evenings a week, plus extra classes on the weekend, all while finishing my training as a nutritionist. Eventually it took its toll and I was strung out, exhausted and ill. I felt broken. I learnt a lot from that year, with the most crucial lesson being how to say no. I had to learn to think carefully, stop the instant 'yes' from escaping my mouth and start to be okay with saying no. Setting boundaries and limitations ensured I wasn't close to burnout, and had the energy and time to give my full attention to the things I was saying yes to.

In my work as an intuitive living coach, I see a lot of women who are like I was then – trying to have it all and struggling. There are too many balls in the air, yet half of those balls don't actually impact their life positively, they simply do them because they feel they 'should'. I find that women by nature find it harder to set boundaries, which in turn means they say yes to being a mother, wife/girlfriend, best friend, colleague, and everything else that daily life chucks on top of them. It's natural to our feminine instinct to be the provider, the mother, the giver, but in order to really be the best in all of these roles, we have to allow ourselves time to reset, before supporting others. Fear of conflict can be huge and women tend to find it hard to say no. We care what people think of us, we want to be the best at what we do, and often have a strong desire to fit in and be seen to be hashtag living our best life. But your success and health cannot be measured on someone else's.

CASE STUDY: JUDITH

Judith was desperate to find love and in the process she was saying yes to everything else, but no to love. She was filling her diary full of meetings, dinners, parties and plans in a bid to keep herself busy and in a position to find 'the one'. But what was clear was that none of this was making her happy and, in fact, it was actually making her exhausted. We worked together to start creating space – for her to sit and breathe and learn how to be on her own without the noise of endless plans. She started to love herself more with all the self-care she was providing her body and mind, but also without realising she was creating space for a man to come in. She did meet someone after a few months of us working together and the tools she has learnt to say no will carry her on through life. It's a joyful story.

When we honour our bodies, time and energy, we are honouring ourselves as a whole. When we find space for ourselves, we find space for our intuition which only enriches its power further, keeping you in your power-zone and flourishing in life. Self-love is knowing when to say no to people, places, food and things, or whatever it is that doesn't feel like it is serving you. It's saying no to things you do not like doing, at times that aren't right for you. It's being healthily selfish and taking time for you. Here's where to start:

LEARN TO SAY NO

As Sarah Knight acknowledges in her book *The Life-Changing Magic of Not Giving a F**k*, you must think about your commitments in terms of energy, time and money. Everything you say yes to, think about how much of these things you are going to have to expend. Question all proposals and give them proper thought. Is it going to be worth it? It is worth your time, energy and money? What does your intuition tell you? Is this the best thing to do? Will this impact your life positively? Will you regret it? Take a look at your calendar. How many things have you said yes to that you really didn't want to do? How many plans did you cancel at the last minute because you had overcommitted and then couldn't follow through? How many times have you overeaten in the past week as a result of feeling pressured by those around you? Next time you get an invite, think ahead as to how you might feel on that particular day. If you know you never enjoy going out on a Monday, don't say yes. If Sunday is your only day to rest and recover from the week, don't book in that 8am yoga class. Don't automatically say yes to everything because you think you should. The biggest thing I have learnt personally is to assess any invite before saying yes or no. As a rule, I rarely make plans on a Monday in order to start my week well with a digital detox and an early night. A polite no is better than a last-minute excuse, so really think about what you're taking on and turning away.

SET BOUNDARIES

The ultimate act of being healthily selfish is setting boundaries. Let's use work as an example, where I find many of my clients feel overwhelmed and overworked! Whether you're self-employed or working for someone else, are you glued to your email after hours? Are you always helping out someone else with their workload and then working overtime to finish yours? Do you never take a lunch break for fear that you'll not get every-thing done? Now let's look at where we get trampled on in our personal life by not setting solid boundaries. Is there that one friend who seems always to need your advice but never appears to listen to it or maybe doesn't return the favour? Is your partner running the kitchen at home and ruling your eating patterns, making you feel out of control or further away from honouring your hunger?

Sometimes there are situations you simply can't control, so try instead to control those you can. Create clear boundaries with both your home and work life. If finding time is a struggle, think about what you can delete from your calendar to free up more of it. Focus on what's important and the task in hand. At work, be honest about your availability. If an employer is expecting the world from you, voice your concerns along with a solution for how you think things could work better moving forwards. At the end of the day you want to be doing the best job you can, and by stretching yourself too thin, this isn't going to happen. Apply the same method to your social calendar and personal commitments. It's time to start setting your boundaries. In the midst of never saying no, you can lose yourself and the ability to hear your inner guidance and intuition. When you can't say no, you are putting yourself in a situation where anger and frustration can kick in – you may feel resentful that you don't have enough time for yourself, or that you are spending time on something you dislike as a result. The to-do list gets longer, meaning the things you love – passions and side projects and self-care – fall by the wayside, which can add to your feelings of resentment. So instead, set those boundaries. Know your limits and learn how to say no when you've reached them.

CASE STUDY: JASMINE

Jasmine had struggled to say no to food. Her husband loved to cook and her social life was hectic – full of drinks parties and dinners. She found it difficult to say no to the endless riches of the foods and drinks offered to her and couldn't remember the last time she felt hungry, truly hungry. Her bowel movements were irregular, she felt bloated and heavy, and her complexion was dry, dull and lacklustre. While she knew she was capable of feeling better, she couldn't gain control through living by her rules for fear of letting people down and seeming a party pooper. But, in turn, she was testing her health and she knew it. Week by week we started creating boundaries and new rules that worked for her. She began saying no to one commitment each week, no to drinking alcohol at one event, and swapped one exotic dinner at home with her husband for something simple, like grilled fish and vegetables. We also looked at how we could make changes to the meals she could control, like breakfast and lunch, creating nutritious meals that would support her symptoms. Each week she took more control and created her own rules, feeling empowered by her food choices and her ability to say no. Within six weeks, she felt lighter, brighter and more in control of her food consumption, plus she enjoyed the feeling of physical hunger on a daily basis.

GIVE YOURSELF PERMISSION

You'll hear me say this a lot throughout the book, but to live intuitively you need to give yourself permission. What do you never let yourself do? If you're in a rut where you're always putting everyone else first and you last, you need to shake things up. Do any of these statements resonate with you?

- I couldn't possibly spend that money on myself.
- I couldn't take that time for myself, what about the kids?
- I shouldn't ask for help, what would people think?
- I can't ask for this time off, I'm the only person free to work.
- I shouldn't eat that cake, it will make me fat.
- I'd love to travel there but I'd feel bad about (insert excuse here).

Let's reframe these:

- I deserve to spend money on myself because I work hard and am nice to people.

- My partner is more than capable of looking after the kids while I go and have some me-time.
- No one will judge me if I ask for help.
- I need to take time off in order to keep myself fully energised.
- I enjoy eating cake – it makes me feel satisfied. By giving myself permission to eat what I want, I never overeat and am in control of my portions.
- Travelling makes my heart sing so I make space, time and money for it each and every year.

Whatever it is, whatever you feel like you'd love to do for yourself but don't, start giving yourself permission. Begin by giving yourself one evening a week, or one hour per weekend, when you can focus solely on yourself. Even if this is a quick bath after the kids' bedtime, take it and make it a priority. If you're a mum who feels you couldn't possibly leave the kids with Dad while you go and get a massage, just book that massage and go, or get someone to come to you. Have you not given yourself permission to laugh properly and you're feeling stern and tired? Go to a comedy show. When it's been a long day and you want to snuggle up with cake and a film, give yourself permission. Start trusting that when you give yourself time and permission, you are honouring your intuition and showing your body that you care. You are making you the centre of your universe.

LEARN TO UNDERACHIEVE

We are all familiar with those days when we just can't finish off that to-do list. By 5pm your brain wants to explode but, instead of ploughing through and pushing yourself to the limit, I want you to learn to underachieve. Personally, I underachieve frequently. I have intentions of getting up early to journal on the weekend and still find myself in bed at 9am. It's the underachieving days that make way for the productive ones. We can't be at 100 per cent every single day. You are all superwomen but even badass women can reach their limit. There will always be times when there simply aren't enough hours in the day, or you don't have enough stamina to get through it. By permitting ourselves to underachieve and championing it – instead of getting frustrated or guilty – we can increase our potential for the next day. Instead of stressing out or feeling over-whelmed, simply ask yourself what the one thing is that you need to do today to have the biggest impact. Do that one task and then give yourself a break. I invite you to say this phrase to yourself the next time you've not managed to tick off everything on your list: 'I underachieved today and it felt great.' Know when you've underachieved and embrace it. Sometimes it really does feel great.

LOVE THE SKIN YOU'RE IN

Is self-love feeling more attainable? Are you starting to create a little love bubble for yourself? In this section we'll be exploring body-love. Hands up who wants body acceptance and a peaceful relationship with food? The reality is we deserve to have both, yet we live in a society that makes it a lot harder than it should be. One of the biggest struggles I see with clients is them learning to love their body, so in this section we focus on body acceptance and how to get it, and body intelligence and how to hear it.

Diet culture is a massive trap. It wants you to degrade your body. It wants you to be afraid of your body. And it's nonsense. Do you want to know the honest truth? People come with a whole range of body shapes and sizes. People who you may consider to have 'flawless' and 'enviable' bodies, which may be fuelling your self-hatred, are often also queuing up to confess their own struggles with food, self-image, body dysmorphia and yo-yo dieting, and the impact that this has had on their friendships, relationships and even careers. Though it might seem like the standards of beauty we have today must be histori-cally universal, this really isn't true. The 'perfect' body has changed constantly over the years, even though the foundation of the female form has stayed the same. The ideal body shape is always evolving; it's never static. What was sexy in the media in 1980 (hello Jane Fonda and her canary yellow onesie) isn't the same as nowadays (here's looking at you, Kim K). What we embrace and aspire to look like today could potentially be at odds with tomorrow's ideal. Now, in the Instagram age, it's clean smoothies and sponsored meal replacement bars, yoga videos and Pilates, all broadcast to millions of followers using #fitspo and #BodyGoals. What we see as the body goal now – slim waist, big booty and boobs – is, quite frankly, more unattainable than ever before. But we have no idea what the future holds.

What I do know is that our bodies will continue to be different shapes and sizes and that women are incredibly magical, knowledgeable and intuitive creatures. Shape, weight and size do not prove worth. There is no perfect size. You are all born unique and should feel powerful and accepted in your skin, whatever shape or size that is. This 'perfect' body is an illusion, so be happy with the body you have and celebrate all the things that make up your gorgeous, imperfect self. I am passionate about helping women to become body positive and love the skin they are in because I truly believe it is the most powerful and revolutionary way that you can understand the strength of your body and mind and, in turn, use your intuition as medicine to heal yourself. Trying to change your body to fit into current beauty standards is unrealistic but changing how you look and feel about your body is real. It's time to embrace the skin you are in.

THE LESS-THAN-PERFECT IDEAL

What ideal are you working towards that makes you feel less than perfect? The real reason many of you aren't accepting your bodies is because of your belief about where you think you 'should' be.

- My stomach should be flatter.
- My thighs should be smaller.

- My boobs should be bigger.
- My bum should be perter.

We associate certain sizes with looking better, being more desirable, and feeling acceptable to ourselves and others. But what if we shook up those beliefs and accepted our bodies anyway? Take away the 'should' and stop defining perfection from the outside in. If we replaced 'should' with 'could' and added 'but I'm happy in my skin as I am' at the end of each of the above statements, it completely turns things around, right?

- My stomach could be flatter but I'm happy in my skin as I am.
- My thighs could be smaller but I'm happy in my skin as I am.
- My boobs could be bigger but I'm happy in my skin as I am.
- My bum could be perter but I'm happy in my skin as I am.

Read these out loud to yourself. Feels good, right? True beauty comes from within. Validation and self-worth must also come from within. You have to reclaim your body and its image as your own. Let's redefine beauty. Beauty is beyond size. Never let anyone tell you any different.

WHAT DOES ACCEPTING YOUR BODY REALLY MEAN?

- It means really being okay and accepting your body now.
- It means wearing a one-piece because that's what you're most comfortable in (even if you think you 'should' be wearing a bikini).
- It means not ever hiding yourself in big, baggy clothes because you don't feel you have the right to be seen. You do. Any shape or size, you do.
- It means looking in the mirror and not seeing every single stretchmark, scar or extra folds of skin as something to be fixed, changed or made smaller.

- Being okay with your body doesn't mean you can't still want to change, but by accepting where you are now and having a kind intention to transform rather than a harsh goal means you are treating your body with consideration, not being your worst critic.
- It means even when being at your heaviest point (hello mums and mums-to-be), you accept your body in a gentle, loving and compassionate way.
- It means having respect for the hundreds of thousands of mechanisms your body performs for you on an hourly basis. You should be internally high-fiving yourself every day.

You have to learn to accept where you are; that's when you can begin to change. You can't hate, criticise and berate your body enough to create lasting change – it just doesn't work. You can, however, be mindful, loving and gentle with yourself and your body; with where you are now on your journey. And be courageous enough not to hide or be ashamed of how you look. Words are everything, and the way we talk to ourselves and to others is important. Here are some of the latest fad memes that we need to stop saying, and why:

STRONG IS THE NEW SKINNY

This phrase is often accompanied by a picture of a giraffe-like creature with long legs and abs so strong they could kill. Yes, these women may be strong on the surface, but are they strong on the inside? I've met lots of 'strong' skinny types who are struggling with the pace of the modern world. Strength comes in many forms, ladies, and just because you don't have a six pack doesn't mean you are not strong. Plus, this phrase makes you feel bad about two things if you are neither strong, nor skinny. Not only that, but I also know a host of skinny babes trying their hardest to gain weight. Which brings us to . . .

THAT PERSON NEEDS TO EAT/EAT LESS

This is essentially 'skinny-shaming' and 'fat-shaming'. We shouldn't be shaming any body type. We shouldn't even be commenting on body types at all. We aren't a label. Neither our weight nor shape defines us. We all have a different body and all bodies should be seen as acceptable to society. Your body. Your rules.

REAL WOMEN HAVE CURVES

Real women have a heartbeat. If you qualify, then you're in! Real women have curves, or they're skinny, or they're big, or they're tall, or they're short. Just because you don't look like the woman next to you doesn't mean she's not a real woman.

BODY NEUTRALITY

The term body positivity started in the 60s to raise awareness of the barriers faced by larger-sized people and as a result, the word 'fat' was reclaimed as a descriptor rather than insult. In the social media age it was re-ignited and used predominantly by women of colour to challenge the beauty ideal. I work with a lot of women who find it hard to relate to the idea of body positivity because it feels too out of reach for them. Here is where body acceptance, or the term body neutrality, comes in. From acceptance we understand that we might not love every single part of our body, but we can learn to accept it. My interpretation of body neutrality is that we should be neutral about all bodies, all shapes, all sizes, colours, genders and everything in between. The more we talk about bodies, the more they continue to be put in the spotlight, sadly opening doors to judgement. With body neutrality we can work towards the concept that instead of emphasising the need to label our bodies, we can

---

learn to make peace with them. My hope is that one day we go even further beyond this, where commenting on how we look doesn't take place at all.

STARTING THE JOURNEY TO BODY-LOVE?

I want you to start thinking about your body in terms of progress, not perfection. And by progress I mean looking at your body, your mind and your soul and how you are growing, developing and living as a whole being. All women are so much more than their bodies. I encourage you to start thinking about your worth linked to your sense of self-identity; your role as a friend, a wife, a mother. Deeper still, your intellect, your ability to learn and have hobbies, your health. Emotionally, your kindness, compassion and your wild heart. These all play a bigger part and have so much more value than mere appearance. A willingness to understand your character, nature and health is commendable and is the first stage in body-love and acceptance. Rather than fixating on the negative aspects of the body, focus on the positives of your body and everything else that you represent as a human being. If we start thinking about attaining perfection as continuous progress, it means we are always working to better ourselves, from the inside out.

Believe me, I know from experience that body-love can be a really difficult thing to cultivate in your life, but I promise that there are things you can do to make the process a whole lot easier! Affirmations are statements that you make in an attempt to alter your unconscious thought processes and reasoning. These statements are bold and full of power which can help to shift your thinking into a more positive direction. Research is beginning to reveal that positive thinking is about much more than just being happy or displaying an upbeat attitude, and that the power of positive thoughts can actually create real change in your life such as increased levels of satisfaction and reduced depressive symptoms.[1] Repeating body-positive affirmations to yourself can help to transform your thoughts and feelings about your body and make you believe what you're saying. I have used affirmations for the last six years and cannot put into words the impact they have had on my mental well-being. I had been searching for a quick fix to lose weight for what felt like my whole life, but when I came across affirmations I found my quick fix to feeling good and a much deeper connection to my intuition through positive thinking. Try using some of these affirmations to cultivate your body-love:

- My body deserves love and respect.
- I honour my body and live with gratitude for all it does to support me.
- I love the way that I look.
- Food is not the enemy and I thank food for nourishing me each and every day.
- My worth isn't defined by my weight or body shape. I define my worth by so much more and I am worthy.
- I love my body, just as I am.
- I accept my body and have thanks for its ability and strength.
- I am comfortable in this skin.
- I accept my body as it is.
- My imperfections make me unique.
- I am confident in my body.

In order to start your journey to body acceptance and positivity, it is time to embrace it. From today you are no longer permitted to downsize, downplay or disrespect yourself and your body. Make a commitment right now to be done with body-shaming. It's over. Start telling yourself and everyone around you that you are good enough and that your body is good enough.

Your body is smart. Your body is beautiful. Your body is unique. Your body is special. As Taryn Brumfitt, director of body acceptance documentary 'Embrace' says, 'Your body is not an ornament, it's your vehicle'. Get behind the wheel and drive wildly into the ride of life.

MAKING SPACE FOR LOVE: THE ROOTED RESET

Rest: Find silence and restore your energy
Reflect: On your relationship with your body and food
Release: The negative voice
Reset: To a new way of thinking

As you go through this book, you'll be learning week by week my tools for eating and living intuitively. For now I want you to prepare by thinking about how you can start shaping a more intuitive you. The Rooted Reset is a guide I have used with clients over and over again, in order to get them to find self-love, body-love and their intuition.

REST: FIND SILENCE AND RESTORE YOUR ENERGY

In our do-more culture nothing is ever enough and rest tends to be the first thing to get sacrificed. It's go, go, go at a pace that speeds faster than Linford Christie. It's causing our minds and bodies to suffer. In many ways our culture considers the body to be inferior to the mind and often teaches us to ignore fatigue, hunger, discomfort and our need for caring and nurturing. It conditions us to see the body as a rival, particularly when giving us messages we don't want to hear. Adverts entice us to purchase products that can banish our symptoms so that we can get swiftly back into the boardroom and the task at hand. This isn't loving our body; rather, it's ignoring the signs it's giving us and so desperately hoping we notice. In order to find self-love and eat and live intuitively, we must first learn to rest. With rest comes stillness for the mind and body to work connectively and, with this fusion, it allows silence. This silence is medicine and using it opens the door to understanding your body's language and, in turn, your intuition.

How often have you worked yourself to the bone before a holiday only to arrive there and get sick? You saved for the holiday of your dreams only to spend half of it bed-bound as your body fixed itself from the year of go, go, go. Start listening to the signals and learn the importance of slowing down. I'm fully aware as I write this that many of you cannot just pop the kettle on, make a cuppa and take five. In fact, I can imagine a few of you are already rolling your eyes at me, as you think, 'I have babies to feed. Bills to pay. A job deadline tomorrow. A nagging child at my knee. Little support. When do you expect me to rest?' Naturally, I understand that many areas of life are non-negotiable and it can be hard to find time, but it is possible to squeeze in small nuggets of rest that can, and will, transform your day-to-day life. By learning how to rest and recuperate, you will recharge your ability to deal with your commitments, your relationships, and your overall health and wellbeing with more energy and more of your feminine force.

THE IMPORTANCE OF REST

Studies show that sleep and rest are essential building blocks of the body and mind.[2] For example, you might just learn better if you take a nap after studying and retain more information long term. You can become stronger more quickly if you take rest days as part of your exercise regime and, when it comes to your body's mechanisms, rest can hugely affect systems from how you digest food to balancing your hormones. Without true rest, we run the risk of triggering hormonal havoc in the body, as cortisol and adrenalin are pumped into the bloodstream – your body in constant fight-or-flight mode. This imbalance can lead to some nasty complications such as depression, weight gain, oestrogen dominance, insulin resistance (stress has a direct impact on your blood sugar levels), chronic fatigue and fertility issues. Worse than all of this is the added stress we pack into an already stressed-out life. By not resting, mentally you are internalising a lot of negativity and losing touch with your own body. The end result is the worst version of yourself – stressed, tired, mentally slow and physically vulnerable, and a far cry from being intuitive.

What if we took some time to look at our symptoms, and why they manifested in the first place? What is our body trying to tell us when a headache is repeating daily? What is our digestive system telling us when we are constipated most days a week? When we look at the physical body, pushing your body into overdrive could manifest physically through a tight neck and shoulders or affect the digestive system, causing symptoms such as gas or bloating. The simple tools that follow are for the time-conscious – my three easy ways to allow more rest into your life.

BREATHE

When you take the time to sit and rest even for a few minutes a day, you are allowing your body to recharge itself on a cellular level (this is why meditation is so powerful). I get that sometimes meditation is not going to be possible, but I challenge anyone to question me in asking you to take five minutes to just be, with your breath. Take a deep inhale through the nose and exhale with a deep sigh through the mouth. You want to try to have a slightly longer exhale here and, if you can, hold the breath after the inhale for a few seconds before you exhale. Just a few diaphragmatic breaths can be enough to rekindle your inner light and find space for silence and your intuition.

BATHE

Your body works so hard for you all day, every day, so the least you can do is treat it like your temple, and give it some time to replenish on a weekly basis. You wouldn't leave your car to run without a service so why would you expect less of your body? Just one evening a week, take time for a long bath in silence. Light a candle, turn off your phone and use lavender or rose aromatherapy oils to get yourself in the zone. Relish the rest and silence.

MINI DIGITAL DETOX

Just once a week I would like you to turn off every single appliance possible, to allow yourself a night where nothing can distract you. Bath night as above might be a perfect way to start this evening (or day if this works better for you), or perhaps you eat in silence and read a book or journal. I want you to learn to be present with your body and mind only. I want you to really zone out of life, and into you. With this book, I am consistently encouraging you to get back into your body. I want you to learn the difference between stretching yourself and overextending – stretching feels a little busy, but overextending feels like you've hit a brick wall. If you can, find other ways to take time to rest. Whether that's a monthly massage or a weekly yoga practice, start incorporating more time for yourself. Nurture your own individual needs and know when to slow down, and when to stop.

REFLECT: ON YOUR RELATIONSHIP
WITH YOUR BODY AND FOOD

Now we've found some silence, it is time to start looking at our relation-ship with our body and food. Reflecting on how we feel about our body and food is the first step in finding self-love and body-love, and living a life guided by our intuition. Throughout this book I'll be guiding you to shift your way of thinking and reject your diet mentality, find satisfaction, feed your soul and make peace with food. To start this process, I ask you to take some time with your journal and reflect on how you have been feeling, your current relationship with food, and how you would like to feel, live and eat moving forwards. This isn't about setting goals but more about your intentions, bringing the feeling into where you want to be with your body and your relationship with food.

Use these questions as a guide:

- How do I feel about my body?
- How do I want to feel about my body?
- What are my issues with food?
- How long have I felt this way?
- Where can I make time for myself?
- What makes me happy?
- What feeling encompasses how I want to feel about my body?
- When did I last have a peaceful relationship with food?

Many of my clients enjoy journalling and reflecting on a daily basis, to document their journey as they go along. Others find taking one hour a week to journal works for them. Wherever you are, start to take time to reflect. It's often wonderful to look at the challenges you've overcome or the goals you've achieved and by doing this you are setting the foundation for the rest of the work in this book.

RELEASE: THE NEGATIVE VOICE

There is much more on this in the next chapter, but for now I'd like you to get into the practice of engaging with your inner voice, understanding the quality of it and releasing anything negative it might be saying to you. The likelihood is we've picked up bad habits along the way and negative thought patterns about our shape, size and food choices have been imprinted on us. In order to eat and live intuitively, we need to practise engaging with our inner voice and releasing anything that is holding us back. This will take five to ten minutes.

Step 1

- Find a calm, quiet space and start to concentrate on your breath.
- Tap into your internal dialogue – what is the quality of the voice? Listen to what your voice is saying. Is it punitive? Harsh? Unforgiving? Or do you offer yourself compassion, forgiveness and kindness? Write these messages to yourself down.

Step 2

- Name this voice. Who is it speaking to you critically? Who is it speaking to you kindly?
- Thinking about the harsh and critical voice, how can it be changed into something more compassionate, kind and loving?

For example, I always found that I was telling myself I wasn't good enough. When I reflected on this voice and where it came from, I realised it had a lot to do with my father leaving when I was young. The effect this had was that I thought he had left because of me. From this, I realised that a lot of the time I pushed people away for not being 'good enough', not because they weren't but because it allowed me to have control of a situation. By pushing my issues back onto them, it meant I could continue to be in control. By pausing and labelling this issue and its origin, I was able to realise how often I was using this voice to control areas of my life.

RESET: TO A NEW WAY OF THINKING

As I've mentioned before, I have worked with affirmations for years and encourage all of my clients to incorporate them into their daily routine. Here is my reset; a very simple, condensed list of affirmations that I love to use when starting an intuitive eating and living journey with a client.

Add in your words and repeat these five times in the morning. This is your reset – a new way of thinking about your body and a new, more intuitive you.

- What word would you like to embody in your daily life?
  (*example:* empowered, authentic, strong)
- I trust myself because . . . (*example:* I'm smart, educated, intuitive)
- Every day, in every way I am getting . . . (*example:* more confident, more balanced, kinder)
- I love myself because I am . . . (*example:* brave, kind, authentic)
- Even though I am not perfect, my flaws make me . . .
  (*example:* unique, brilliant, interesting)
- I can do anything in life because I am . . . (*example:* smart, brilliant, bold)
- When I look in the mirror I see . . . (*example:* love, a woman, strength)

SELF-LOVE: THE TOOLKIT

Aside from the tips I have given you throughout this chapter, here are my go-to tools for your self-love toolkit; simple rituals that bring you back into your body and back in love with yourself. You might like to try all of them, one of them or none of them, but I encourage you to try them all at least once. We are all different and what works for some may not work for others. Find what does work for you and roll with it. Give yourself time and dedication. Remember, this is all for you and there is no right or wrong way.

START YOUR SELF-LOVE JOURNAL

Over the past decade, there has been a huge amount of research to show the great social, psychological and physical health benefits that come from giving thanks. I want you to start giving thanks to you. Studies have shown that gratitude had a strong direct effect on body appreciation, and body appreciation accounted for a large portion (88 per cent) of gratitude's relationship with intuitive eating.[3] Each evening, start reflecting on what you feel gratitude for from that day. It can be a simple list of five things or a stream of consciousness – again, there are no rules here. Try to go for depth over breadth; elaborating in detail about a particular thing you are grateful for carries more benefits than a superficial list of many things. Savour surprises and try to record things that were unexpected, or spontaneous. Don't try to overdo this – it can often be a quick five lines before you head off to sleep. Other days you may feel like giving yourself an hour. Then, whether it's daily, weekly or monthly, start to write down why you love you. As a guide, maybe ask yourself some questions such as: What are your positive traits? What's great about you? Why do you love yourself?

TAKE CONTROL OF THE SCROLL

I'm going to let you in on a little secret. Instagram is not real life. Social media has its benefits, but it's also a quick way to beat ourselves up and a comparison trigger for us to think that everyone has it sorted and is living a better life than us. This is NOT true. Start to recognise the people, Instagram accounts, tabloid papers or daily newsletters that appear in your inbox that, quite frankly, make you feel a bit shitty about yourself. Stop reading up on celebrities if you feel like you'll never measure up positively to them. Unfollow your friend from school who seems like she has it made and prompts you to compare yourself to her on a daily basis. Take control of the scroll and determine what you want and don't want to see.

MIRROR MIRROR . . .

Who is the fairest of them all? You are. Start looking at yourself in the mirror and talking to that incredible vessel of yours. You can begin with clothes if you need to, but work up to staring at your naked form. I want you to start doing this as often as possible, ideally once a week minimum. For every negative thought you have about your body, start to counteract it with a positive. For example:

Negative: I have cellulite.
Positive: I have strong legs.

Negative: I hate my stretchmarks from being pregnant.
Positive: My stretchmarks are the signs of my womanhood and I
    am proud to have a beautiful, healthy baby.

Negative: I hate my bum.
Positive: My bum gives Kim K a run for her money, and it's natural!

Negative: I hate my boobs.
Positive: My boobs are beautiful and soft.

Start to see your imperfections for what they are – a part of your story. Turn every negative thought about your body into a positive and tell her. Connection is life force and it starts with you.

THE POWER OF TOUCH

I'm big on touch. In recent years, a wave of studies has documented some incredible emotional and physical health benefits that come from touch. Research shows that touch is truly fundamental to human communication, bonding and health.[4] Just 20 seconds of touch releases oxytocin, a powerful hormone that acts as a neurotransmitter in the brain. It regulates social interaction and sexual reproduction, playing a role in behaviours from maternal–infant bonding and milk release to empathy, generosity and orgasm. It has also shown to increase generosity in humans.[5] Skin on skin nurtures us emotionally with feelings of trust and connection, but when was the last time you touched your own body with the intention of love and kindness? You have to start touching, looking at and seeing your body in all its glory in order to love it. Start by massaging your toes in the bath, and then move up on to massaging oil into your belly and thighs. Stroke your own neck or learn how to do a facial massage. By generating a sense of connection with our skin, we can learn to hear how the body signals to us. Later in this book you'll see how important this is in connecting with your intuition.

MEDITATE

This is my favourite meditation. The goal is to switch on the acceptance button in your brain. Start by slowing down the breath. Close your eyes and inhale and exhale deeply to start the journey within. Close your mouth so you are only breathing through your nose. Filter incoming air and breathe more slowly and serenely. Become still. The only thing moving is the air coming in and out of your body. Observe your breathing and how it flows. Is it short and sharp, or long and calm? Can you slow it down just that little bit more? Inspect your emotions from the outside. How is your mood? How is your body feeling? How are you feeling? Try to breathe as slowly as possible. Imagine your breath bringing light and positivity into your body and taking out any darkness and negativity. If you are troubled by thoughts, sounds or sensations, simply recognise them as you inhale and release them on the exhale. Bring your attention back to your breath. Think about the miracles that happen every day. Thank life for these miracles. For our body, our life, our abilities. Every day is a day to be thankful for. Now go through the affirmations below. Just read the words and repeat to yourself, bring the affirmation into your body and smile within.

- I choose to have goals in life but also to remain flexible and open to the surprises that life has to offer me. I say yes to things I want and need and no to those that do not serve me.
- I cultivate kindness to my body, and by doing so I also cultivate self-worth.
- I welcome the opportunity to step out of my comfort zone and I do not let myself be guided by fear.
- I trust in my intuition and trust that it will be my greatest guide.
- I accept myself unconditionally, because it is essential to my happiness. I accept the person I am and I do not need other people's approval to accept myself fully.
- I am going to respect my body and give it the nourishment it deserves by drinking water, eating fruit and vegetables, walking and exercising. Today I am giving respect to my body.
- I try to be impeccable with my words, and speak to myself and to others only with positivity.

Start to take a slightly deeper breath. As you come out of the meditation, slowly bring awareness back to your senses and into the room.

Well done, you've made it through the week. Are you feeling loved-up with yourself yet? Continue to work on that love bubble over the coming five weeks. Now that we have laid the foundation for self-love, in the next chapter you are going to learn how to tackle your inner critic. It is this critic – or toxic self-talk as I like to call it – that often gets in the way of using your intuition.

You Are What You Think

IDENTIFYING TOXIC SELF-TALK

Are you aware of the voice in your head? The one that bosses you around and tells you what you shouldn't or couldn't do? Yeah, I know her. She is part of what the girls at Project Love call the shitty committee – they stop you living your best life. I call mine Neggy Nancy. This inner voice provides a running monologue, sometimes cheerful and supportive and sometimes negative and defeating. This chatter is your self-talk and sometimes she needs to learn to take a back seat. As my mother used to say, if you've nothing nice to say, don't say anything at all. If only Nancy lived by this mantra. Listening to what your intuition is telling you will always bring you back to peace and clarity, but when the inner critic is keeping your internal negative monologue loud, it can be hard to hear your intuition through all the noise. This is what we are exploring in this chapter – how to tune in to your inner critic; the concept of the inner child and how this can govern your inner critic; how we understand the critic and reshape it, making it a BFF and not an enemy. We'll also be delving into where our diet mentalities and body blocks have come from and how we overcome them to find a place of even more self-love and body-love.

Your self-talk combines your conscious thoughts with your unconscious beliefs and biases. It's a very effective way for your brain to interpret and process your daily experiences, both good and bad. Unfortunately, it's human nature – especially when it comes to our bodies and our ability and appearance – to veer towards negative self-talk, or toxic self-talk as I like to refer to it. These pesky comments might start out as a whisper, but eventually they can become a roar and that's when this negativity becomes unrealistic and can be detrimental to our health. Your thoughts are the source of your emotions; the food that fuels your mood. They influence how you feel about yourself and how you respond to events in your life. But when we delve a little deeper into this concept – known as mind–body medicine – we understand the ways in which emotional, mental, social, spiritual, experiential and behavioural factors can all directly affect health.

The concept of the mind being important in health and illness dates back to ancient times. In the West, the notion that mind and body were separate entities began during the Renaissance and Enlightenment eras. Since then, increasing numbers of scientific and technological discoveries furthered this split leading to an emphasis on disease-based models, where all too often we treat the symptom, and not the cause. When illness strikes, we have learnt to pop a pill. Belief in the mind's role in health and illness began to re-enter Western healthcare in the twentieth century, led by discoveries about pain control via the placebo effect and the effect of stress on health. I'm not asking you to believe that the placebo effect can cure illness, but what I am encouraging you to do is explore and be curious about how your thoughts, feelings, beliefs and attitudes can negatively affect your biological functioning. A study of female students, published by the Psychology of Women Quarterly, found that 93 per cent of the women involved were engaging in this toxic self-talk, with a third doing so on a regular basis.[1] Their findings indicated that those who complained about their weight more often were likely to have lower satisfaction with their bodies – irrespective of their actual size.

A campaign that I come back to time and time again in explaining the power of positive affirmation and self-talk to my clients is one from IKEA. They partnered with an advertising firm, Memac Ogilvy, to show the effects of bullying on plants and brought in students from a local school to take part in the experiment. Two plants were given exactly the same food, water and light but one plant was played recordings of positive affirmations such as 'seeing you blossom makes me happy', while the other was played polar opposite statements such as 'you look rotten'. It is not surprising that the plant that was exposed to only negative comments turned brown and began to rot. While some may doubt the science behind this experiment, it offers a little insight into the tremendous impact words can have on us, and this is what I want you to explore in this chapter, and ongoing.

The power of words is in your hands or, literally, in your head. Every time you speak negatively to your body, it senses it and absorbs it into your cells, muscles, tissues and organs. The more negative the thought, the deeper it goes. When directed to specific parts of you, it doesn't just stay there. Why? Because these organs work together to perform a function and these functions work together to build a system, such as the digestive system or respiratory system. It's a ripple effect.

Words do matter so be mindful of the fact that your cells might be listening! Try this for yourself by observing the way in which you talk about your body and, in turn, how it responds. When you tell your body it's fat or ugly, it's bound to feel stressed and vulnerable. You tell her she's strong or beautiful and she'll want to sit up straight and show her strength. Read these to yourself and think about how the words feel in your body:

- You are ugly
- You are disgusting

- You have too many wrinkles
- You are fat
- I don't like you

Now read these to yourself and think about how it feels:

- You are beautiful
- You are smart
- Your skin is clear
- You are magical
- I love you

Hands up who preferred round two? It's not hard to see how a derogatory choice of words can have a negative impact. Consider how you feel when someone compliments you. Whether it's your outfit, your new hair, your ability at work or your infectious laughter, you light up. Now imagine how you could feel if you complimented yourself on a daily basis. You can learn to challenge and override your negative self-talk and, like all habits or changes you want to enforce, the first step is becoming more aware of it.

Scientists studying the inner voice say it takes shape in early childhood and persists as a lifelong companion. In my practice with disordered eating and body positivity, I've come to see this as true; it can often be the cries of your inner child, the echo of the child you once were. It's here that your self-esteem, body image, family trauma and shame reside. Everyone has their own unique history, influenced by their environment, events and significant people. Many of my clients have picked up negative self-talk from memories and experiences imprinted on them from their childhood. They will often need guidance to reconnect with their inner child, talk to it, nurture it and assure it, and ultimately re-route it down a more positive path. When it comes to emotional eating, time and time again I see it emanating from a deep desire for approval, something that perhaps was longed for as a child. This connection between our inner child, our adult self and our relationship with food is easy to understand when we consider that, as babies, our first experience of being comforted is when we are being fed in our mother's arms. Your inner child stores many of these memories, and the impact they had. What you picked up about body image and associations with food from childhood may stick with you for life.

> This relationship with your self-talk is intimate and constant.
> It is the most intimate relationship you have.
> It is the most important relationship you have.

For many, their toxic self-talk is not in fact the voice of a tyrannical dictator but that of the scared little child living inside them, playing dress-up like an adult yet trying desperately to have their needs met. Acknowledging and nurturing the inner child relationship with the self is critical to better body image, self-love and living more intuitively. It determines the degree to which your mind and body are connected. Here's how to identify whether it could be your inner child directing your self-talk:

- Your parents separated during your childhood
- A parent had a disordered relationship with food or body image
- Your younger self struggled at school
- You have a sibling who you always compared yourself to
- You were ignored as a child
- You were bullied as a child
- You have a co-dependent parent

This is not a definitive list. Your inner child might have had a different experience or a combination of those mentioned above. Here are some examples of how an inner child might be controlling the adult you, your decisions, and why:
- You are a people-pleaser (this often comes from always trying to

please parents, or not feeling good enough as a child)

- You are a control freak (this comes from something happening to you as a child that was out of your control, such as parents breaking up, the trauma of losing someone)
- You can be aggressive or frustrated easily (this can come from being frustrated as a child – perhaps by too much control from your parents or siblings)
- You look for approval when making decisions (this often comes from not trusting in yourself as a child – you tried to use your parents, teachers and friends as your inner GPS)

INNER CHILD

Allow me to share my own journey with the inner child, and perhaps you'll be able to identify with any similarities to your own, or it will trigger memories from your own childhood. My father left when I was young and then wasn't consistent in our weekend visits, cancelling at the very last minute, often that morning. My mother couldn't allow him to treat me in this way. A toddler, excited to see Daddy, only to be let down at the last minute. Before long, I didn't see him at all. My mum was a grafter and worked her socks off to keep me, my brother and sister afloat. She had a day job and worked part-time at night, so I was often looked after by my older siblings, nannies and childminders. What else could my mother have done? Of course, none of this was intentional but, for an impressionable child, this was the first example of what a relationship with a man should be like. When I was seven years old, my mother remarried a man who had two daughters, one of whom was a friend of mine from school. It was a lot, learning to share my mum, and it took a lot for me to transition to having two new sisters. I also moved into their house, which meant making friends with their gang. They had been friends for years and I always felt like the outsider in this kids' group. It's only looking back that I realised this and my father's behaviour had shaped a deep desire for approval. I longed to be loved. I took to food for comfort but, as I grew up, the desire for approval evolved into wanting to be thin, which would, I thought, make me more desirable. And so began the bingeing and purging. I would weigh myself every morning, after school and even after a poo. If the scales showed an extra half a pound, I would spiral. My world revolved around food, and my weight.

Growing up, I took to parties and a longing to be loved by men. I wanted everyone to love me, because I didn't love myself. It felt easier that way. I was the life and soul of the party and that identity felt good. But it wasn't me. It was only when I eventually identified (with the help of my therapist) that it wasn't adult Pandora making these decisions, but poor vulnerable inner child Pandora longing to be loved, that I started to be able to take control. As a way to have this need met, I had created the Pandora I thought I should be, one that people would love and adore as my father hadn't. It was a false self – an ego whose sole purpose was to please. I began to connect with my inner child. I talked to her daily. I told her she was loved. Over time, she became my BFF and we walked together in life; we still do. By reducing the people-pleasing and learning to love myself, I started hearing my intuition and what it was guiding me to in life. I allowed myself to be led by it. What once was a career in fashion and beauty PR turned into training to teach yoga and study nutrition. I started feeling real. I became my authentic self.

So here you see how our conditioning often comes from our upbringing. We are shaped by many things in life. I'm not saying that there is blame to be placed, just that an understanding of your inner child and any deep-seated wounds is important when working through any barriers that are stopping you from connecting and living with your intuition. We need to come to this understanding without blame or judgement. Our parents were on their own path and we ours. We can only learn from our journey to become our most authentic self.

What makes you break your diet, or run up your credit card, or be attracted to all the wrong people? You know these aren't healthy things to do and much of the time you know you're sabotaging your own best interests, but it feels a bit uncontrollable – sometimes you just can't help it. Sometimes there's no reasoning with the bold beast on your shoulder! Could that be your inner child calling the shots? We all have self-sabotaging tendencies and these behaviours are attributable to a part of our personality that needs to be acknowledged and accepted. Maybe you didn't even know you had it? Well, now you do.

The relationship with your inner child is the most important relationship to nurture. If you want to get comfortable with living a life led by intuition, you have to get comfortable with living openly with your inner child. You have to get comfortable with you – your adult self – and your inner child, walking hand in hand through life together. While everyone experiences their own individual upbringing, I see patterns emerge among my clients when they describe issues around food and body image. These are explained below in three types:

THE ABANDONED CHILD

This inner child usually manifests as a result of parents divorcing or being too busy to spare attention. As a result, this child feels lonely and insecure and, in order to offset such feelings, they use food as comfort.

THE REBELLIOUS CHILD

This inner child was controlled in varying forms throughout childhood. Whether it was a controlling parent or strict schooling, this child rebels with food. Cue eating chocolate for breakfast.

THE FEARFUL CHILD

This child is likely to have received a lot of criticism and, thus, never felt good enough. In a bid to experience love, they use food to quite literally bring on the feeling of fullness – and feel 'enough'.

You may resonate with one or all of the above but by identifying the child that still lives within you, you can think about what that child actually needs right now. Would you give her food if she was hungry? Would you tell her to shut up, toughen up and stop crying? Or would you sit with her and hold her, giving her the attention that she needs? Try to give your child self what she is calling out for. Try to send some compassion to the part of you that feels abandoned, rebellious or fearful, but which is just trying desperately to have her needs met. Think about what you needed as a child but you didn't get. How can you give it to yourself? Here are some of my favourite tools to connect to your inner child.

JOURNAL WORK

If the inner child concept resonates with you, take a moment to write down in your journal three ways in which you think your inner child might be holding you back or calling the shots. Underneath, write why you think this might be happening. Note: This is not something to be afraid of. As soon as you embrace your inner child, you'll find a freedom in understanding a little more about yourself. With this freedom, you'll find a little more peace and you'll be able to discover your intuitive wisdom.

REKINDLE YOUR RELATIONSHIP

You are at one with your inner child; there is no separation. Reconnect with your inner child by making a list of things that brought you joy when you were young. Explore these memories; that childhood wonder that kept you pure and youthful. Revisit activities you loved as a child, such as colouring in, running in the woods or playing dress-up. What else did you love doing as a child that you no longer do?

WRITE A LETTER TO YOUR INNER CHILD

Once we've reconnected to our inner child, we may find we have so much more to say to find peace with them. Simply writing a letter to your inner child to apologise or expressing your desire to reconnect can be powerful on the road to recovery, leading you to self-love and inner wisdom. Tailor your letter to the type of inner child you have. If she is fearful, reassure her. If she is rebelling, tell her you honour her freedom.

CREATE A SAFE SPACE FOR CONVERSATION

Your inner child is vulnerable and needs protection. By creating an open space, you allow feelings to be felt and emotions to be explored. I encourage clients to create space for their inner child daily. Whether that is physical space or by wearing something like a necklace or ring that you can touch and connect with daily, you are quite literally allowing space for your inner child to be heard and feel safe. When emotions surface, try to identify whether it is adult you feeling them, or your vulnerable inner child.

CASE STUDY: MEGAN

Let's take a client of mine, Megan, whose mother was anorexic and whose family were very judgemental when it came to bodies and how people 'should' look. Megan was constantly engaged with thoughts about being slim along with a deep need to rebel against her mother so as not to become her. She was in a perpetual cycle of bingeing and then starving, over and over again. Her world was riddled with thoughts that she needed to be better, stronger, smarter. In a bid to manage these endless thoughts and to be 'the best', she became a counting control freak. Calories, macros, micros were one thing, but Megan also had a desire to be the best at everything. She was jealous of anyone who was smarter or skinnier, and when she didn't feel like she was the best, comparison controlled her and she would obsess about the result or person over and over again. She controlled everything in her life and it felt overwhelming and exhausting. I helped Megan identify that this was not adult Megan controlling, it was her inner child speaking, who was so scared of being judged on how she looked and what she achieved.

While adult Megan wanted to move past her family's ways of thinking, inner child Megan was stuck there, feeling abandoned and alone. I gave Megan a gentle lead into acceptance and flexibility. First we looked at speaking to her inner child daily, telling her that she was accepted, safe and that she wouldn't be judged. Then we worked on an acceptance piece, accepting her mother's illness and how she had grown up, and rewrote her own story instead of her living in her mother's. Then we addressed where we could create more flexibility in her life. Her goal was to find freedom with food, so Megan stopped reading food labels, created new dishes each week, and ignored all forms of counting devices, from Fitbit to the scales. Over time, Megan stopped seeing things in such an all-or-nothing way; she stopped comparing and, most importantly, she started living *her* story. She and her inner child were no longer stuck in the pendulum of disordered eating and control, and instead created flexibility and freedom with food, her body and her mind.

STORYTELLING:
THE DIET MENTALITY REVEALED

Though the inner child concept may have resonated deeply with many of you, there are other reasons why our self-talk can become toxic and this is what we'll be exploring in this section: the idea of storytelling and the impact it can have on our thoughts and feelings. We'll look at the layers of stories and mentalities that you may have built up in your subconscious, fuelling your toxic self-talk and clogging up your ability to be intuitive.

We live in a world of storytelling. From national news to chats in the local with Bob the barman, we all have a story to tell and we all deserve to be heard. Unfortunately, in our share-more culture, we've become accustomed to taking on these stories as our own, or as a comparison guide to how our lives should be lived. All stories and experience have an effect on us and, whether we've picked them up from family, friends or the media, they are absorbed deep into our subconscious and have a direct impact on our inner critic. When we are only listening to our inner critic, our intuition is hard to hear.

INVITING YOUR SELF-TALK OUT

Take a minute to shut your eyes and connect with your self-talk. Sit, breathe and be with this practice. I encourage you to start checking in with it on a daily basis, listening to the quality of it and what it is saying. Don't fight it, just be aware of it. The more you learn to recognise and listen to this inner critic, the easier it will become to understand where it is coming from, whether that be your inner child or other stories and imprints you have picked up on the journey we call life. As humans, we crave connection and so the more you can connect your mind and body, the more you will feel at one and at peace with your body. When you can master positive self-talk, you can become more confident, body positive and happy. You can think yourself to live intuitively. Here are some pointers to ask yourself:

- Think about what you've said to yourself today.
- What did you tell yourself about how you looked, what you should eat or how well you performed at your job?
- Now where did this voice come from? You or your inner child?
- Now tap into the tone of this voice. Was it critical and harsh? Or was it kind and compassionate?
- Think about how you felt after you engaged in this inner discussion. Was it a one-way conversation? Were you fighting back and telling the inner critic to do one?
- Deeper still, where in the body are you holding your emotions and this self-talk? Does it come from the niggle in your shoulder? Or the constant rumble in your tummy?
- When it came to a diet mentality and body image, did your self-talk order lunch for you? Did it critique your food choices and your body?

While we can't always completely detach from the stories we encounter, we can learn the art of non-attachment. It's not always you directing the toxic self-talk; it's often the stories and perceptions and opinions of others that you've picked up along the ride of life and taken on as your own. So many women live their lives governed by 'shoulds' that they have never really thought to question. Many things you have always considered to be absolute truths are nothing more than socially constructed norms – hoops that we are taught to jump through or ideals we are told to live by.

Let's look at where some of your mentalities and blocks could come from. We live in a world that is riddled with guilt around everything from food to our carbon footprint. It's a world which for many feels full of comparison. While social media has its benefits, it has also created an opportunity for us to – as comparison coach Lucy Sheridan calls it – compare and despair. Social media, by its darkest definition, offers a filtered peep into the lives of others, fuelling our perception that our own life isn't good enough. Health-focused memes and slogans (no pain, no champagne) that on the surface bring a smile are actually loaded with judgement and a mentality that says, in order to look great, you have to work hard at the gym, be strong not skinny, or put your body through a process unattainable to so many yet unanimously desirable. Then we have the saturation of information in the modern age. Dr Google, blogs, 'experts' without a qualification – when it comes to diet and 'healthy eating', it's becoming harder and harder to know what to believe is good for us. Under the guise of health, we are struggling more with disordered eating. We have more information than ever before, but we've moved further away from knowing what is right for us individually. We've stopped listening to our bodies.

As far as our bodies are concerned, and how we feel about them, almost no one escapes unscathed from the trap of consumerist culture, which creates an insatiable desire to change ourselves. It's all around us – eat this yoghurt and become a goddess; drink this product and meet the man of your dreams; use this shampoo and you'll reach orgasm in the shower. Industries exist to gain money by conditioning us to believe that the way we look or the way we are is intrinsically wrong. Great for those companies making the big bucks, but not so good for us, the vulnerable consumers. It's time to wake up to your beauty and feed your body with the love and tenderness it truly deserves. As a society we think and talk about body image and food (especially dieting) in moralistic terms – good or bad. Think about how many times you've heard, 'Ooh this is such a naughty dish' or, 'I was really good until dinnertime and then I ate bad foods.' When you dine with friends, do you judge the one who can eat anything she wants? Or maybe you think you shouldn't eat certain foods because Linda next door said she lost seven pounds when she stopped eating them and secretly you hope that it might work for you too. That's

Linda's story, not yours. What works for her body might not for yours. I'm pretty sure this is an experience you can relate to, even within the last week.

Looking specifically at food – breakfast, lunch, dinner, snack – who made up these rules? Yes, there are many nutritionists out there who attest to the importance of breakfast, plus science to back it up, but if you are someone who feels physically sick from eating before 11am, surely it's a sign it's just not right for you, and your body. There should be no rules when it comes to your own food consumption. How often do you have days when you just want to eat; you're ravenous from morning to night? Then there may be days when you wake up and simply don't feel like eating. This is your body telling you what it needs and every day will be different to the next. Tune in and make your own rules, which we'll come to later in the book.

All of these cultural influences and imprints have informed our own journeys, but when we begin to question these truths – whether we have internalised them through our own personal and family histories, or through societal and cultural norms – we begin to wake up. This process can be painful but also beautiful and incredibly life-affirming. It only leads you closer to your authentic self, and living with your intuition.

CREATING A FILTRATION SYSTEM

To live intuitively it's important to create a story filtration system to help us understand what is really our truth, and what thoughts and beliefs we are carrying around that are not our own. Start to identify where your food mentalities, body blocks and other attitudes around your ability in life have come from. Who is it that's talking to you when you think about your body or food? Who or what is it that is limiting you? Rejecting these blocks and mentalities allows you to shift the ideals that you have been presented with in the past about how you should look, your weight, how you should feel about your body, and even how you should live. Throw out the books, magazines, people and social media accounts that offer you false hope when it comes to your body image or that restrict you from being your authentic self. Look around you. What adverts, social media accounts or people are causing you to reject your own sense of self or keeping you thinking small? You are in control.

Now let's go deeper and identify how your toxic self-talk has been playing tricks on you by overruling you with limiting mentalities. It's time to let go of anything holding you back from eating and living intuitively, time to create a new story that is more positive, balanced and sustainable. You can overcome these mentalities by reframing and reprogramming your brain and replacing old beliefs with new ones. Here's how:

- Take your journal and find a place to sit quietly.
- Start to engage with your own diet mentalities and body blocks.
- Try to identify where they have come from. What comes up in your body? What is your mind saying? Write it down.
- Now think what there is about this mentality that you can release in order to get you thinking more positively.
- Now, what do you accept in order to find peace around your mentality?

Here are some examples of blocks and mentalities I see the most:

Block: To be desired, I should be a certain size.
Where this came from: Comparing my weight to my sister's.
I release: Comparing myself with the body of others.
I accept: My body and weight as they are.

Block: I don't deserve to eat what I want.
Where this came from: Being restricted with food as a child.
I release: The idea that food should be restricted.
I accept: That all foods are neutral.

Block: The body I want is unattainable.

Where this came from: Trying to look like someone else.

I release: Negative thoughts about my body.

I accept: My body as it is.

Block: Eating what I want will make me fat.

Where this came from: A fear of not being on a diet. Dieting keeps me safe.

I release: Fear of food.

I accept: I can trust my body.

You can use this tool for any blocks, from your career to relationships. So much of the time we are programmed to believe our life 'should' be lived a certain way, yet what I find with the women I have worked with is that this usually isn't their story but one they have created based on others. They have taken opinions and stories and made them their own. Can you start to reject others' perceptions of reality and start listening to your intuition? Stop denying yourself your heart's desire in order to fulfil someone else's. Stop with the 'shoulds' and 'should nots' when it comes to decision-making. What do you desire and what could you achieve? Know now that you are on your path, creating your story. You are the centre of your universe.

GETTING OVER OVERTHINKING

The opposite of intuition is overthinking and it is one of life's many soul-suckers. In this section we will look at why we overthink, how it manifests and how it sucks the life out of us. Are you a control freak? Do you have a deep desire to know all of the answers? Are you never able to let things just be? Do you find yourself out of sorts if things don't go to plan? Do your irrational thoughts busy your head at night? If you answered yes to any or all of these questions, you are letting overthinking and control rule your life. And it's time to change. You aren't alone in this. We are inundated with choices and information. Much of our stress today is caused by overthinking things. We have identified that we cling onto stories but we also cling onto control, scared to drop anything we might be juggling. It's only natural that we overthink. We live in a world rich in information and science has led us to a desire to know the answers to everything. We often have an intense desire to be in control all of the time. We leave very little room for the imagination or the notion that it simply is what it is. Sometimes we have to let go of understanding, and allow things to just be.

Overthinking can be life-leaching. Consider the number of times you have spent time and energy thinking negatively about something and allowing it to take over your mind, not to mention your evening with family or friends. Or perhaps you're a scenario overthinker who goes over and over how a situation might pan out instead of just being open and welcoming any result. The outcome is not trusting in the natural course of the situation. Overthinking can rob us of happiness and who has time for that? Not me. There are a few ways I believe overthinking destroys your ability to think and be intuitive. Can you relate to any of these?

Overthinking:

- Keeps any problem a problem. You keep yourself stuck inside the same problem until you quit thinking about it and either find a solution, or let it go.
- Often makes situations worse. Cue taking a problem from work home with you, only to let it affect your family life too.
- Prevents your creative problem-solving skills from bubbling up. You spend so much time thinking about the problem, you forget to think about the action that is needed to overcome it.
- Makes you worry, and worry is nothing more than your imagination creating a further negative state of mind.
- Sucks your time and stops you from being mindful – you're so busy

in a past or future negative state of mind that you completely forget about right here and now.

- Robs you of energy that could be better focused on things that are worthy of your attention.
- Leads you to second-guess yourself and creates self-doubt.
- Creates heightened negative feelings like anger, resentment, jealousy, fear, doubt, indecision and confusion.

When we have toxic self-talk with thoughts that aren't based on reality, it's called cognitive distortion. Cognitive distortions are simply ways in which our mind convinces us of something that isn't really true, usually taken from the stories we've been fed or imprints from our experiences, including those that are not our own, such as from friends, family or the media. Inaccurate and exaggerated, such thoughts create chains and patterns that have a knock-on effect; continuing to reinforce negative thinking or emotions. These negative beliefs then fuel toxic self-talk and we continue telling ourselves things that sound rational and accurate, but in reality only serve to keep us feeling bad about ourselves and unhappy in the skin we are in. Here are some examples of the cognitive distortions I see most often in my clinic:

- Personalising – taking something personally and seeing events as your actions. There is always a bigger picture.
- Mind-reading – guessing what someone is thinking, when they may not be thinking that at all. This is useless.
- Predicting negatively – always thinking of the negative outcome first and underestimating your ability to cope with it. Trust that the future can be bright!
- Entitlement beliefs – believing the same rules that apply to others should apply to you. They don't.
- Seeing a situation only from your perspective. There are two sides to every story!

- Recognising feelings as causes of behaviour but not equally how this behaviour influences thoughts and feelings, such as 'when I have more energy, I'll exercise', not 'exercising will give me more energy'.
- All-or-nothing thinking – for example, 'if I don't lose seven pounds, I'm a failure'. You're not. Buy some new jeans and love your body as it is now.
- Shoulds and musts – for example, 'I shouldn't eat that.' You could, though. Try it!

Here are a couple of examples of cognitive distortion with regard to a diet mentality and body block:

Fear: If I stop dieting, I won't stop eating.
Reality: Dieting is often the trigger for overeating. You starve yourself or constantly diet, and then inevitably you pile the pounds back on when you reach for the pasta dish and face-dive straight in. You've starved your body and it rejected you. Once your body learns and trusts that you won't be starving it anymore, the intense need to eat and binge will decrease. Your body will feel satisfied, full and complete. You yourself will be satisfied.

Fear: To be successful or loved, I must be thin.
Reality: Nobody can be the expert of you and your success and nobody determines how you yourself can feel loved. Who determines your success? Do you love yourself? Only you know your abilities, your goals, your money mindset and how to expand and reach nearer towards them. Only you can define success and allow love in. Your weight does not define you, or your ability to be loved.

As you can see, these fears and the reality are so far apart. Your fearful thoughts are in the UK and your reality is down under in Australia.

Cognitive distortion is at the core of my work with intuitive eating and living where I see endless clients who live in a world riddled with fearful mentalities, none of which are their own but all of which need untangling.

Another way in which overthinking can be negative and make you feel bad is linear thinking, such as thinking only of the goal – the end point – and not about the journey. When you are focused on something, for instance how much weight you are going to lose, you are thinking about the end point. Inevitably, when this goal isn't achieved or takes more time than expected, you may feel you've underachieved or, worse, like a loser. To live intuitively is to live the journey, not the result, so instead of linear, try switching to process-thinking. Instead of setting one end goal, try thinking in terms of small steps. Instead of aiming for one great leap, try focusing on continual change – the learning process – one baby step at a time. Instead of looking at every deviation, embrace everything as a learning experience.

CASE STUDY: NAOMI

Naomi, a young woman I mentored, had a mind full of cognitive distortion. She believed she had to be thin to be successful, that if she gained weight she wouldn't be beautiful and that she wouldn't be loved. She was uncontrollable around food and, as such, would have complete binges, many of which she would barely remember. These binges were quickly followed by feelings of guilt. She came to me to find some answers about why and how she had these thoughts so often and to help her find a place of balance with her body image. It turns out that Naomi had a very controlling father and, as a result, her upbringing was full of restriction. To accompany this, her father was controlling of her mother's weight and would make remarks if she so much as gained a pound. It was clear that Naomi's inner child was that of the rebellious child, constantly trying to rebel with food as a way of gaining control. As for the cognitive distortion, the comments her father had made to her mother had become so deeply imprinted that Naomi truly believed that if she gained weight, she wouldn't be loved. When Naomi and I unpicked her cognitive distortions around her body and food and replaced them with a harsh piece of reality cake, she started to be able to manage her binges and, soon, stop them completely. We connected her to her inner rebellion and assured her that she didn't need to take such action anymore. She wouldn't ever be restricted again. She was free.

OVERTHINKING: MIND AND BODY

Where are you holding stress? Where does it manifest in your body? What weight is on your shoulders? Is this weight your own? Take a body scan now, and consider what you are feeling in your body. This development of awareness depends on breaking through places in the subtle body that may be blocked with unresolved issues and energy.

In yogic philosophy, there is no separation between the mind, body and spirit. The three exist as a union; one definition of the word yoga. This philosophy believes that what happens to the mind also happens to the body and spirit, and so on. In other words, if something is bothering you spiritually, emotionally or mentally, it is likely to show up in your body. When your body is blocked, you may be unable to detect the subtle feelings that your intuition is giving you. Though the ancient yogis understood that emotional turmoil is carried in the mind, the body and the spirit, Western medicine has been slow to accept this idea, but new research has verified that a person's mental and emotional condition can affect the state of their physical body, and that the mind–body connection is real.[2]

As you work deeply with your body in exercise such as yoga, emotional issues are likely to come up and be released. In fact, anytime you work with the body, you are also working with the mind and the energy system, which is the bridge between body and mind. This is why we tend to hold a lot of trauma in the body when we've had a stressful period or even a stressful day. Overthinking can affect your ability to be free in your body and, if you aren't free in your body, you aren't free in your mind. I always encourage clients to do gentle bodywork daily to encourage any stagnancy to be released. Time and time again I see clients who feel like there must be something wrong with them but tests prove differently. When I ask them how they are emotionally, they'll explain that stress causes them to feel like their stomach is in knots. This sensation is the evidence of stress impacting the body, due to the two being interrelated.

The secret to living intuitively is to stop trying to control the chaos of life, and focus on what you can control – your own actions, words and thoughts. There is no one stress-free life, just like there is no one perfect body. Simple, everyday, focused activity can be the solution to ease a busy, stressed-out life. You do not need a hammock or a beach in the Bahamas to live life stress-free, but you do need to take control and find space for moments of joy, relaxation and stillness throughout your day. The continuous practice of these mini moments of calm and stillness counterbalances the stress response of fight or flight – your sympathetic nervous system – which prepares the body for something intense, like vigorous physical activity or an altercation with a sabre-toothed tiger. Many of us are living in this state of high intensity – driven by the sympathetic nervous system. Of course, none of us is about to be chased by a tiger – or at least I'd hope not – but modern life means we are living a high-stress, busy and sometimes chaotic existence. The more we learn to engage with our parasympathetic nervous system – which has almost the exact opposite effect by relaxing the body and inhibiting or slowing many high-energy functions – the more we can find the mini moments of calm, and feel more in control of the chaos.

LETTING GO

When overthinking takes over and is causing you to feel stressed, panicked or anxious, you can learn to direct your energy using positive intention and action in order to create a new habit of calm. You can't press 'pause' on the world and slow down the challenges of life, but you can be aware of the mind. I call this finding silence and using this as medicine. In order to find this silence, we must learn to let go. By finding silence we can feel more in touch with our intuition; we can allow it to be heard. In this silence we find calm. Here are my failsafe ways to reduce overthinking:

CHECK YOURSELF BEFORE YOU WRECK YOURSELF

Before you can begin to address or cope with a habit of overthinking, you must first become aware of it. Next time you sense you are spiralling into overthinking, stop and check yourself. Try to acknowledge it and check in with yourself. How much time and energy is being consumed? Are you behaving passively, instead of actively? Realise that thinking once, or just a few times is enough. It leads you nowhere rethinking the same thoughts over and over again. Make a decision to be aware and act by giving yourself a time limit of five minutes to think about the situation, and then write down all the things that are worrying you, stressing you, or giving you anxiety. Let it rip. Let it go! When five minutes are up, throw the paper in the bin and get on with your day.

DISTRACT YOURSELF

Walking, swimming or exercising the body in any way can temporarily take your mind off the habit of overthinking. Anything that keeps your mind occupied with some activity that doesn't allow you to overthink is okay. I find a quick walk around the block helpful and not too disruptive to my working day.

RIGHT OVER WRONG

So often, our cruel nature leads us to automatically think negatively about a situation. In many cases, overthinking is caused by fear: fear of the outcome, fear of not being in control, fear of failing. Don't think of what can go wrong, but what can go right. Take control of the situation and visualise all the positive outcomes that could occur. Better yet, visualise the outcome you want and then list the actions needed to get there. Accept that you will give your best in the situation at hand and that no one can predict the future. But by combining faith and action, we might just be able to direct the outcome.

CHANGE YOUR VIEW OF FAILURE

I once read a meme on Instagram from a business coach which read, 'There is no room for failure.' I wholeheartedly disagree with this statement because you know what, we learn so much from our mistakes. Things you've been fearful of in the past will be different from what you fear now. If we've failed in the past, we've learnt something from it and it doesn't mean it will happen again. There is always a learning in every process. There is an opportunity with every new beginning. What can you achieve today?

GET PERSPECTIVE

This is a big one. How bad is the situation? When in the process of overthinking, catch yourself – are you making a mountain out of a molehill? Ask yourself how much this will matter tomorrow, next week or in five years. Just using this simple question and changing the timeframe can bring a fresh, new perspective.

STOP WAITING FOR PERFECTION

Step away from the control button in your brain. For all of you who are seeking perfection, you're waiting at a bus stop for a bus that was never built. There is no 244 to perfection city. Ambition is admirable but perfection is unrealistic, impractical and debilitating. The moment you start thinking that a situation needs to be 'perfect' is the moment you need to remind yourself that waiting for perfection is never as smart as making progress.

CREATE A RITUAL

To make any process of letting go official, you can simply sit still with the intention of releasing the event from your consciousness. As you do so, you allow it to be present one last time, you honour it with your attention, thank it for teaching you, and then kindly guide it on its merry way. Imagine the thoughts leaving your mind and body – out the door, out the window, out the top of your head, or into the earth through the soles of your feet, liberating you from the burden of them. Allow yourself to feel lighter.

Reduce overthinking
Move forward
Make mistakes
Trust your intuition
Find your purpose

When you break up with overthinking it's like creating your own 'get-out-of-jail-free' card. It gives you a free pass to end your relationship with the drama inside your head and it will free up space to focus instead on things in the present and hear your intuition as a guide. How do you feel about overthinking now? Can you see how it might have stood in the way of hearing your intuition? How much of your overthinking can you let go of to make space for the here and now? It's calling but will you answer?

OVERCOMING COMPARISON

There is nobody else like you in the world. You are truly unique. Did you know that? I'll tell you again, you are truly unique. I tell you this because just like overthinking, comparison robs you of precious time by letting your self-talk run wild. Too much self-talk means too little time to hear your intuition. Comparison is another of life's soul-suckers, and it's one that has the ability to go on, and on, and on. There is an infinite number of categories to which we can compare ourselves and an almost infinite number of people to compare ourselves to. Once we begin down the rocky road of comparison, we run the risk of never finding the end and we can become truly lost. In this section we look at comparison and how to beat it.

We get 86,400 seconds each day and using even one of them to compare your body, accomplishments or life to another is one second too many. We have nothing to gain from comparison, but a lot to lose: passion, drive and self-worth to name a few. Comparison is always completely unequal; typically we compare the worst we know of ourselves with the best of others but, frankly, we are far too unique to compare ourselves fairly. Think about it – you can't possibly compare yourself to anyone else because your own gifts, talents, successes, contributions and value are entirely unique to you and your purpose in this world. It is human nature to want to see how we measure up in comparison to others – especially if we think that they are better than us or have more of something that we want. And of course it's the world we live in now that has created this comparison bubble.

I'm Generation Y – born in 1985 – a generation that was the first to dabble with the digital world that we know today. Anyone born between the early 1980s and early 2000s – millennials – lives life predominantly online. I remember the days when your friends would know what you did on the weekend based on what you'd tell them on Monday morning at the school gates. Now, they would know from my constant stream of updates on the various platforms I express myself on: Instagram, Facebook and Twitter. By the time Monday came around, they'd have seen it all anyway. Don't get me wrong, I love social media and the connection and opportunities it has brought us as a generation, but I'm also fully aware of the dangerous side of the digital world – one where we can become plagued with comparison to others.

It started with a bit of oversharing on Facebook and the ability to see what your ex was up to. Now we've got to a point where our Instagram feeds need to be picture perfect – a pristine, polished image or perfectly posed snap to post alongside our carefully worded caption. Sadly, social media provides us with numerous platforms which can trigger unpleasant self-disdain. It allows us to see into the world of others through their highlights reels, while we struggle with insecurities behind the scenes. Every time you look at someone's feed, you are only getting the very best aspects of their lives, which, in turn, can make you feel like your life, by comparison, isn't as good. Seeing the best version of everyone else's life can make you feel deprived. To top it all off, we have the number of likes we obtain from our posts, which just like taking drugs, drinking alcohol or smoking produces dopamine in the body; the chemical associated with pleasure.[3] No wonder we are all addicted to our phones!

We all know that gut-wrenching feeling when we see or hear something that immediately has us second-guessing our ability, appearance or personality. Comparing yourself to others will ruin you. It kicks you when you're down and ends your goals before they've had a chance to start. You could compare yourself to your boss who has the position you want, earns more and, therefore, has the bigger house and wears designer clothes to work. For years you grind your way to the top, you reach the level of the boss, but by this point they have their own company and have moved to LA to live their dream life. And so the process starts again. Who do you compare yourself to now? Your boss is living his or her life, and you should be living yours. The good news is that, just like overthinking, we can take control of our comparison.

One of the first questions I ask my clients when focusing on body image is, 'What's stopping you from feeling good in your body?' An answer I invariably get is that they compare themselves too much with others. It will often take me the whole first session to explain the client's choice of words. They don't even realise how much they are comparing to their sister, mother, Kim K or Sheila from down the road who manages to get to the gym every day. They'll believe that these people must have a better life than their own because they make it to Fitness First by 8.30 every morning. For many of my clients, the root of self-loathing, body-shaming and unhappiness is comparison. They compare everything, from their bodies to their social status, car and house size to their handbag collection and everything in between. They aren't alone.

I remember as an innocent young girl being obsessed with being the prettiest, the smartest, the 'best'. Growing up, I looked at other girls' bodies with intensity, always striving to find out what made the 'perfect' physique, how they ate, what they did to look like they did. I'd secretly stalk women in the gym, watching their workouts hoping to find 'the secret' to the perfect body. How I wished someone had told me back then that I'd never be the best at anything and that perfection didn't exist. The world is far too big for that. The truth is that when it comes to body image and living with purpose, it is not a good use of time to compare ourselves with others because there is no one like us and this makes us incomparable. When you make a judgement on others, and compare yourself to their ability or appearance, much of the time it is a mirror facing back at you. What you see in other people can be a reflection of yourself.

Let me ask you this: when you compare yourself to others, is it that you don't feel good about what you have and who you are? Does the grass seem greener in your neighbour's garden because maybe, just maybe, you're pissing on your own lawn? Or are you looking at theirs from a distance, scared to create a lawn like it for yourself? It is sometimes easier to look outside of ourselves and feel like we are deficient in comparison to other people than taking responsibility for our own progress. It takes a lot of courage to look within to see whether we are measuring up to our own standards or meeting our own full potential. Are you living your purpose? Are you satisfied? To compare our lives to other people's when we have no idea of what they are here to learn or fulfil doesn't benefit anyone – especially you. This is an important process on the path to self-acceptance and eating and living intuitively. If you are comparing your body with someone else, what are you resisting in your own?

I'm too busy working on my own garden
   to notice yours is greener.

Comparison gets in the way of you being you, as you try to be everyone else and everything in between. To overcome the battle with self-love and body positivity, we have to overcome comparison. Each of you has special gifts, a unique body and genetic make-up. You each have a life purpose to fulfil and with this come the lessons that you must learn and the experiences that you must go through in order to evolve as spiritual beings. You must expand and explore your own path, not someone else's. Your individuality is worth celebrating, rather than searching for faults and comparing your uniqueness against anyone else. Instead, begin to accept yourself, appreciate the vehicle you were given at birth, as well as your incredibly special talents and qualities. Then you will quickly realise that everyone is going through certain kinds of experiences for a reason and you can become less focused on what other people have or are doing. Realising and valuing your uniqueness enables you to bring out the best in yourself, so you can get on with living, rather than preoc-cupying yourself with meaningless comparisons. Try to not compare yourself to others, and you will see how much you have and how special you are. Focus on you, you and only you.

HOW TO OVERCOME COMPARISON

The solution to the 'grass is greener' attitude is practising self-appreciation. Self-appreciation involves both staying off other people's lawns and focusing and taking care of your own! Overcoming comparison requires focus and tools such as taking control of the scroll, as described in Week 1. Only you can take control of what you see, so if someone or something is fuelling your comparison, unfriend and unfollow: the power is in your hands. It is our own filters and comparisons that get in the way of us being able to see our uniqueness and our ability to shine.

DON'T LABEL YOURSELF

Comparison often cheats us into thinking that we have to be the same or fit into a certain perfectly sized box. If you're unsure of exactly what your path is or your purpose, or even what you want to have for your tea, it's okay. Perhaps you can't sum up who you are, what you want, or where you're going, and that's okay too. Don't allow comparison to keep you feeling stuck; it's okay to break out of the box and take some time working on what path you're on. On your way, you'll experience what you need to, and maybe even learn a new way and connect with yourself in the process. Be you and walk your own walk.

APPRECIATION LIST

When you're feeling particularly frustrated, jealous or hopeless with comparison, stop, breathe and write out a list of things you appreciate about your current situation. In doing so, you bring the focus back to yourself; you have enough and do enough already. And when you do decide to get or do more, it will come from a positive, healthy, loving, inspired place instead of a dark, negative and unhealthy bottomless pit.

COMING BACK TO YOUR STORY

When you come across something that makes you compare yourself, direct your mind back to the idea that you create your own story. This mental exercise will quickly alleviate any anxiety produced by comparison and put you back in your garden with your lawn, on your soil, with your own blossoming potential. Repeat this to yourself over and over:

- By focusing on self-improvement – personal progress and not perfection – rather than comparison, I create a more realistic and insightful approach to living intuitively.
- I keep showing up for myself.
- I trust that I am destined for good things and that good things take time.
- Authenticity is everything.

How do you feel now at the end of this section? Are you ready to quit comparison and allow space for your own intuitive life? Remember that no one person has it all. Everything you want to create and feel is within you. Now that the inner critic has been identified and you've learnt how to notice when the comparison button gets hit, we are going to look at shifting into a new way of thinking.

PROGRESS, NOT PERFECTION

Here's a secret for you – perfect does not exist. The infinite amount of information in the modern age when it comes to diet, body size and 'healthy eating' means that nobody knows what to believe. What I do know is that you can be healthy and beautiful whatever size, weight or shape. I do not believe that you have to be thin to be fit, happy or loved. In this section I'm introducing you to seeing things differently;

health and your body in a new way. You are so much more than your body. What is most beautiful and rich is being real. From today, I want you to start thinking about your health, mind and body as progress, and not perfection. Focus on your journey and not the destination. With progress you can look deeper into your abilities, your connection to the mind, the journey to a kinder, happier, more intuitive you. Are you ready to progress?

Your body is just a form of you. If you lose an arm or a leg, you're still you; only your physical body would change. When we are constantly shaming our bodies by talking negatively to them, we are reinforcing the idea that there is only one shape or size that is beautiful or perfect. The expectation is that we 'should' all have the perfect body but the reality is that there is no set perfect anything: no perfect world, no perfect life, no perfect body. You only have to look at your family and friends around you to know that we are all shapes and sizes. The idea of perfect is subjective. Perfect is an illusion that no one can attain but progressing – whether that's in learning to love your body or learning to eat intuitively – is possible in a much more manageable and sustainable way.

I want you to think about what identity means to you. What do you think about yourself and your identity? Where do your family, friends, hobbies, intellect and health sit? Do you want to be valued as kind, vibrant, interesting? What's your 'why' in life? What does your bigger picture look like? These all play a key role in your identity, with a much higher value than just your appearance. How are you progressing as a person, a woman, a soul? If we start thinking about progress and not perfection we learn to think about the bigger picture in every situation. What ideal are you working towards that makes you feel less than perfect? I've expressed before the value of the relationship you have with yourself; it's continuous progress – always working to better yourself, from the inside out. The reality is you are all perfect just as you are. To live intuitively allows for progress; a deep understanding that every day will demand a different you. How beautiful is that? The more you learn to live intuitively, the more you can be flexible in your progress.

One of the reasons we aren't accepting of our bodies is because of our belief about where we think we 'should' be: my stomach should be flatter; my thighs should be smaller; my arms should be more toned; my butt should be shapelier.

We associate certain sizes with looking better, being more desirable, and feeling acceptable to ourselves and others. But what if you shook up those beliefs and accepted your body anyway? What could life look like then? To fully appreciate your body, your health and your life, you have to ignore what others think of you, what others have, and what others do. Only your thoughts influence your happiness. You can change your thoughts but you can't change theirs. One of the most effective ways to switch from striving for perfection to working on progress is that of 'reframing'. Reframing shifts our thinking about a situation – an event or a mindset – and teaches us to form a different perspective. It teaches us to look at failures as learning opportunities. This process allows us an expanded view of our reality and the power to see progress in everything. Here's an example:

> 'The best way for me to lose weight and have the perfect body is to follow a strict diet and exact eating plan and weigh myself each day.'

What we are seeing here is a very specific mindset; control and a heap of internal judgement. With reframing we take the negative and turn it into a positive. This practice helps you to first identify how you might be unconsciously holding a diet mentality or body block, and then offer you a more positive and flexible approach. Such as:

> 'There is no perfect body or diet and using strict eating plans takes me further away from eating intuitively. I can trust in my body's hunger and fullness signals and allow myself to choose foods that I find satisfying. The scales give me false information and affect my mood.'

JOURNAL WORK: REFRAMING

Note down how you perceive yourself when looking in the mirror and how you feel about yourself and your body. If any of the testaments are negative, work on how you can reframe them into something positive. Create positive self-thoughts that counteract your negative and potentially damaging ones. If you're thinking pessimistically the whole time, why? Write it down. Can you reframe these thoughts to be more optimistic? Look back on your day – did you focus on failing to make the gym rather than highlighting the few days when you felt good about your body and smashed that 5k run? Here's an example of a belief that connects our feelings towards ourselves and food:

'I don't deserve to eat whatever I like.'

Is that you? If so, try reframing to something like this:

'I'm a worthy human being and deserve to get pleasure, satisfaction and nourishment from my eating experiences without feeling any guilt.'

The only opinion in the entire universe that is of importance to you is your own, and your opinion affects your entire life! Replace your complaining with appreciation. Think about your wins rather than your losses. When we stop defining perfection from the outside in, we realise that true beauty comes from within, as do validation and self-worth. You have to reclaim your body and its image as your own. Beauty is beyond size so start to redefine it. Be happy with the body you have and celebrate all the things that make up your gorgeous, imperfectly perfect self.

GOODBYE INNER CRITIC: THE TOOLKIT

In identifying how you speak to yourself and learning how to let go of any toxic self-talk to make more room for your intuition, there is going to be a mourning period. You are going to have to come to terms with the fact that the critic is gone. To finish this section, here is your weekly toolkit to confront, recognise and reject the inner critic. In dealing with the death of Nancy, there may be a grieving process. Just like mourning a partner or a pet, you may feel abandoned, fearful, angry or depressed. She's going to try to return but, like any toxic relationship, you have to be strong and trust the process. In shedding Nancy's darkness, you are only making space for light. I've worked with many people who have taken to their new voice with ease. Others have needed a little more guidance. In doing so, I ask them to speak to themselves as they would their best friend. It's time to make your self-talk work for you. Here's how:

THE NEW NANCY

Give your new positive self-talk a name. This might be your inner child or someone else; you decide. Move over Neggy Nancy; you have the ability to create a new Nancy. This person is your biggest fan. They adore you, big you up, challenge your self-doubt. Language matters and your words have power. Hear your new Nancy roar.

START SMALL: TAKE THE ONE-WEEK CHALLENGE

Challenge yourself to a week of no toxic self-talk or body-blocking. It might be hard at first, but set the intention to get through each day with kindness and love. If you need to, tell your friends and family about it so that they can support you. If it's those around you who are driving the toxic talk, tell them you're bored of body talk and alert them to the negative impact of their words – for example: 'I adore you and it hurts me to hear you talk about yourself that way.'

FOCUS ON THE FUN TALK

Avoid discussing diet and exercise and instead focus on how you are feeling. Replace words such as fat or thin with vibrant and energised. With anything diet-related, from food choices to your food shop, start to think about the emotional and health benefits. So, if your friend has started a new fitness regime, instead of asking about weight loss, perhaps ask them whether they're feeling stronger or sleeping better.

REPLACE NEGATIVE WITH POSITIVE

If you start to fall into the body-talk trap, use the reframing tool and try turning the negative into a positive. Think of a positive replacement state-ment for everything negative you might say about your appearance or that of others.

For example:

> I shouldn't eat this.
> ~ I can eat this but I will only eat until I am full.

> I'm too fat to wear this.
> ~ I embrace my shape and wear what I feel good in.

> I will be stupid at that fitness class; everyone will look at me.
> ~ No one is looking at me and I will feel great afterwards.

TACKLE YOUR HARSH WORDS ABOUT OTHERS

As I've explained in overcoming comparison, what we see in others is often what we see in ourselves. If you're judging someone on how much they are eating, their choice of clothing or their body, hair or skin – what is this saying about how you feel about yourself? Check yourself when you start thinking about critiquing others. Stop yourself if you feel the urge to criticise other people's weight or looks. Take a long, hard look at yourself and how you might actually be judging yourself. Observe the situation – what is this experience teaching you?

YOUR NEW STORY

Your journalling tool for this section is a powerful one. When I started my own healing journey, banishing Neggy Nancy was important but, without her, I felt like I was living in a grey area. It's important for you to start creating the new you and get clear on how she feels about herself, her body, how she eats and drinks, and the woman she is.

Set aside 30 minutes and write down in your journal:

1. What your goal is
2. Your daily commitment to get there
3. What you need to release to get there
4. How you want to feel

For example:

1. I want to cultivate positive self-talk
2. Spend one minute telling my body all the things I like about it
3. Judgement
4. Empowered

You can then turn it into a daily journalling practice by writing down affirmations based on your new story. For example:

I am a woman who ... only speaks positively about her body.
I am a woman who ... doesn't judge.
I am a woman who ... gives time to talk to her body.
I am a woman who ... feels empowered in her body.

This process helps you clarify what you want for your body and self-talk, but you can take it further into life too. You need to identify what is in your way in order to work on releasing it. Sometimes it can be something emotional, spiritual or a physical block; sometimes it can be another person, or even a place. Use this process to stop thoughts going round and round in your head and, instead, brain-dump – pen to paper! Relax into it, allow yourself to see the way forward. Allow yourself to see the new, more intuitive you.

We will never live our legend if we are constantly following someone else's script. Rejecting that negative voice and listening only to positive words and our desires as if they're a road map to our truth is the way we as women live our uniqueness. It's how we live with intuition. Each of has a unique voice the world deserves to hear. The key to unlocking it is to cherish your own story and your place in it – feel powerful, feel alive and feel abundant. We are all impacted and influenced by others – we can't escape that – but what we can escape from is the negative effect, which should never be held in our body or our mind.

Now you have built self-love and tackled your toxic self-talk, you are ready to really connect with your intuition. Welcome to Week 3: listen to your body.

Listen to Your Body – Understanding Intuition

What is Intuition?
Your Great Power
Seeing the Signs
Listen to Your Body
The Power of Trust
Identity: An Intuitive Life
Intuition: The Toolkit

WHAT IS INTUITION?

Intuition is:

- The ability to understand something instinctively, without the need for conscious reasoning.
- A thing that one knows or considers likely from instinctive feeling rather than conscious reasoning.
- A 'gut feeling'.

You've met with the foundation of this work in Weeks 1 and 2 and now we are at Week 3: understanding intuition. I'm thrilled for you to be here and learn more about living intuitively and what it offers for your relationship with food and your life overall. Just as learning self-love is about being your own BFF, finding connection with your intuition means you get to spend time with and feel the support of that BFF every day.

As a child, I remember being called 'emotional' a lot. I was the cry baby, the thinker, the sensitive one. It's only through this work that I realised the emotional side of me was one of my biggest strengths: my inner voice, my gut instinct, my intuition. No wonder I loved and still do love being alone. I enjoy my thoughts and my silence, because it's here that I connect with my intuition. Intuition or using your intuition isn't the magical phenomenon that you may have been led to believe. There is a lot of talk about what intuition is and I myself – before I started this work – thought that to be intuitive was to have the ability to speak to the spirits and the dead. I imagined Whoopi Goldberg in the film *Ghost*, in her candlelit room, shiny gold dress and a crystal ball. Little did I know. This chapter helps you to clearly understand your intuition, connect with it, strengthen it, and confidently follow it.

ARE YOU INTUITIVE?

Let's begin by seeing if you are in fact intuitive. Answer yes or no to the following questions:

1. Have you ever had a dream?
2. Can you see?
3. Are you able to hear?
4. Can you think of something that has happened in the past?
5. Can you visualise in your mind's eye the beach and a deep-blue sea?
6. Do you have memories?
7. Are you breathing?

If you answered yes to any of the above, you, dear reader, are intuitive and in full possession of your intuition. To be instinctive is to be guided to action or to do something without conscious thought. Living with our intuition is a process that gives us the ability – a tool – to know or feel something without analytic reasoning, bridging the gap between the conscious and non-conscious parts of our mind, but also between instinct and reason. We've all heard of women's intuition, but men have it too, although research suggests that women are, as a sex, more intuitive. One study[1] used MRI scans to compare male and female brain connectivity and discovered that the typical male brain is neurologically wired to be more logical, and thus more effective at linking perception with action. The female brain, on the other hand, was found to have more neural connections, making women better at interpreting social interactions, such as facial expressions, tone of voice and body language. Women are more likely to pick up on subtle emotional messages, as well as to express their own emotions and be more empathic. It's being open to these emotions, both what people are thinking and feeling, that gives women the ability to be more intuitive.

In the same way that we have a digestive system, a cardiovascular system and a sensory system, we all have intuition. It is a tool that we are born with and no different from any of our other senses. You won't have been educated on intuition at school and yet it is a natural part of who we are. I can bet most of you have experienced gut feelings that you can't explain, such as meeting someone new and knowing that you're going to make friends instantly, or simply loving or hating a new property when house hunting. Some of us are born with a stronger connection to our intuition, while for others it takes a little more work. But this is similar to some of us having a stronger digestive system, or higher muscle-to-fat ratio. Though we all have the same components, we are unique in the *way* we are made up.

Intuition is the communication tool you have between you and your spirit, or soul. Just like you may concentrate on the gut for healthy digestion, you should be focusing on establishing connection to your intuition in order to find true health and alignment. For this section I want you to use your journal every day. In each section there will be a focus point – something I want you to connect to in order to connect deeper to your intuition. There will be a lot of practical work, so how you use this section is up to you. If intuitively some things resonate with you more, practise these tools more. I am simply giving you the information, and want to encourage you and inspire you to try this work for yourself. This is your creative power. That's the beauty of intuition – it is a point of power; a tool for creative expression and for the expression of your personal power in our world.

INTUIT: TUNE-IN TOOL

1. Write down an example of when you have used your intuition and then have a question in mind that you would like your intuition to guide you with.

2. Lie down and get comfortable. Allow the breath to come deeply into the chest, and flow out calmly through the mouth. Allow yourself to feel the support of the floor below you. Breathe into how that feels. Feel it deeply. More deeply. Deeper still. Relax for a few more minutes, then, when you feel the urge to get up, say internally to yourself, 'I will allow myself to relax for a few seconds more.'

3. Now, let's allow your intuition to provide information. Stay as you are or sit up. Ask your higher guidance: 'I trust my intuition will guide me with . . . [insert your question].' Sit and wait. Wait and watch, listen, and allow the answer to come. Allow also for the possibility that no answer will come, but that's okay too. Just allow it to be. Don't judge or try to create what you think the answer is, just be. Write about your experience in your journal.

YOUR GREAT POWER

So the big question you might be asking me is: how exactly do we connect with our intuition? In this section we look at how to develop a relationship with your intuition, how to follow it and most importantly how to trust it. Many of us live in a fear-based culture that is obsessed with trying to control life. We're terrified of uncertainty, so we're constantly anticipating everything that might go wrong and doing everything within our power to guard ourselves against inevitable disaster. But in doing so we aren't allowing life to just flow. You don't need fear to protect you because you have your intuition, a potent, trustworthy compass that will guide you to your true path.

Think of life as the world with many roads, and you as the traveller driving a car and exploring. You have your body and mind in the car and you have a programmed GPS. Sometimes you take the wrong turn or go off-piste to find a better route. Sometimes this route is turbulent and you might have some troubles along the way, but you get there in the end. This GPS is not angry when you make mistakes; it just keeps searching for the shortest and safest way to reach your destination. This GPS is just like your intuition; it's there to guide you from A to B. When you tap into your intuition, that GPS is guided towards the right direction. If we don't listen out for it, we might end up taking the wrong turn.

Everything you need is within you. Because intuition is our spirit's language, it speaks in many voices and appears in many forms. Sinking into the silence to hear it was my biggest lesson in life. Being a people-pleaser, I was the queen of keeping myself busy. A do-do-do, go-go-go mentality meant I barely had time to think about my needs, which kept me safe. Being with my own thoughts felt incredibly lonely – a place where I daren't go. By learning to slow down the pace, step outside of my comfort zone and into my power, I began being more and more guided by this inner GPS. I promise that all of these tools have been tried and tested, not just by me but by the many women I have worked with over the years. Some of them may resonate with you, others not so much. I dare you to try them all out regardless. I often find that it is the tasks and tools we resist the most that are the ones we *need* the most. Whether it's physical healing, relationship help, or financial guidance, intuition works, so allow it. Here's how to start tapping into your intuition:

REWIND

One of the easiest ways to get to know our intuition is to rewind and look at the times when you ignored it. Have you had moments when you knew you were staying in a job or relationship for the wrong reasons? Or times when you felt pulled to a decision but fear got in the way to keep you safe? Maybe you regret certain situations due to not following your gut instinct. Allow yourself some time to reflect on these. What pulled you away from your intuition here? Hindsight can be useful to help us interpret the signs intuition is giving us and how we can work to trust it more in the future.

SLOW DOWN

Take a deep breath. Continuing the process of Week 1, where can you find some time for yourself to be still? For those of you who have a tendency to pile more and more on your plate in a bid to stay busy, work up to this by first taking five minutes a day to do nothing but be still. Then work up to a longer period. Can you manage a bath without listening to a podcast or some music? Turn it off and be with your thoughts. Then this could turn into one evening a week, maybe up to two. We are always communicating internally but how is your ability to hear from within? Learn to really listen to that voice, that small, still voice.

USE YOUR SENSES

Whenever you want to listen out for your inner GPS, it's important to feel your feet on the ground, be aware of your hands, and be able to listen to the room around you. This helps you to drop into your body. Using your senses is the most powerful way to feel into your body. Taste, touch, smell, sight and hearing are the gateway to your body.

Close your eyes and take a few deep breaths. Find access to your body and your intuition through your senses. Start noticing all that you can with your five conventional senses. Doing so allows you to access your sixth sense.

MEDITATE

Messages from your intuition tend to be quiet, so spending time in silence will help you to hear and interpret them. Meditation allows us to connect to a higher state of consciousness, and communication between the conscious mind and the physical body is dramatically enhanced. Meditation is a simple, effective way to tap into your internal dialogue. It slows the mind, calms the breath and relaxes the body. Meditation helps develop your intuition in several ways. By clearing your mind of any recurring worry or stress that plagues you, it allows you to hear your inner voice more distinctly and louder. Meditation will also teach you how to slow the fast pace of your mind and to exist in the present moment. When you are free from the burdens of fear, worry, stress and uncertainty, you can then reach the place where your intuition grows and evolves. Likewise, intuition stems from the right side of the brain, which meditation helps to develop and stimulate.

LEARN THE ART OF SELECTIVE HEARING

One of the most important ways to connect to your intuition is to allow selective hearing. Do you remember when your mum would say, 'I feel like it goes in one ear and out of the other'? Well, it might just be that you had learnt the magical art of knowing what to store, and what to stop! By this I mean what you're letting in and out of your mind. Do you hear all the negativity and fear-based talk from your colleagues? Do you feel emotional after watching the news? Do you have a friend who is critical of your every move? Don't allow those sounds to fill your mind. Who and what are you exposed to can have a huge impact on your ability to thrive, be positive and listen to your own inner guidance. I encourage you to let go of anything you find negative and draining, by literally allowing these comments to go in one ear and out of the other!

DREAM BIG

Allowing yourself to daydream is a playground for intuition. Daydreaming merges the conscious and the subconscious minds, and since intuition is largely a subconscious practice, daydreaming can serve as a gateway to invite both worlds to dance together.

Ask yourself the question: 'What makes me feel alive?' Take some time to allow your mind to consciously wander in answer to the question. Notice where your thoughts take you and go where they go. You may have something specific you're wishfully thinking about – a holiday, new lover, a new job in a new city or country. Allow your imagination to take you there. Be guided by your inspiration and creative, spontaneous self. A big part of why I love connecting to daydreaming and dreams as part of intuitive practice is that they can also be fun, as you let yourself focus on something that isn't constrained by everyday conventions. You can use this to your advantage by daydreaming about a subject or problem in an unusual way, and then writing down the results. It might just inspire you to find a new method for creating something or solving a problem, one that perhaps wouldn't have occurred to you in your waking, organised world. It might just get you thinking differently, inspiring a wider vision, solving a problem or creating your magic! I find daydreams can also get clients into alignment; by quite simply giving yourself time to sit and reflect, you are giving yourself time to focus on your life. Magic can come from being aware of your dreams and daydreams.

A NOTE ON YOGA

This isn't a book on yoga but I must emphasise the impact of yoga as a tool to develop your intuition. For me, yoga was *the* game-changer. It cultivates your intuitive abilities and allows for a deeply spiritual experience. It helps you to understand your body and the subtle shifts that take place which can have a big impact on how you think and feel. Our body has an intuitive way of protecting itself by tensing certain areas under stress; we tighten the hip flexors, neck, shoulders and jaw, to name a few. The physical practice of yoga flushes out any stuck stress energy that accumulates from old injuries, toxins stored in our cells, or emotional baggage. By learning to make safe and positive decisions for our body in the moment of yoga, we can identify and release this resistance and tension, intuitively making choices that ultimately serve us, not just in body, but in life.

Mentally, yoga allows us to experience stillness and, in turn, cultivate space to hear the inner guidance of intuition. Just like our body, our mind doesn't want to be tight or weak. In yoga, we activate and communicate with all parts and systems of our body and mind, as opposed to searching for answers outside of this sphere. Typically, we often seek connection through outside sources, such as social media, people or the television, allowing both our heart and our intuition to be drowned out by the voices of others. Yoga helps us to quiet these voices so we can find answers from within. As we learn to turn inward, we cultivate our intuition, our instinct and our intelligence.

Yoga also works on the emotional body by releasing old wounds, tensions, stresses and strains. It teaches us to feel, to be more present with our emotions and label them as they are experienced. For some of you, the practice of yoga may be a challenge, for others already a part of life. Whether you're mustering the courage, finding time to practise daily, or haven't even considered yoga to be a part of life, the biggest hurdle to reaping the rewards yoga offers is getting on the mat. It's difficult to imagine what will happen once you start practising yoga, but you won't know until you do. Wherever you are, I encourage you to explore.

There will always be times when you struggle with doubts about whether the hunches you have are really your intuition or whether you're just making them up. Wherever you are on this journey, make a conscious effort to develop and use your intuition. You never know where it might lead you.

SEEING THE SIGNS

Now that you've learnt the tools to connect to your intuition, let's explore how your intuition might be speaking to you. Open your eyes wide, clean out your ears and listen deeply. Your intuition speaks in many ways.

WHISPERS FROM THE UNIVERSE

When your intuition tries to communicate with you, it may give you gentle nudges in the right direction by prompting you to notice little patterns; it's like it's trying to get your attention. I call these whispers from the universe; intuitive messages, gut feelings or informational downloads that seem to come out of nowhere. This can happen in the form of subtle guidance or feelings. For example, if you've been thinking about finding a new job but have been sitting on the fence due to limited beliefs in your ability, you might notice a job posted by a friend on Facebook or something advertised in your local paper. Alternatively, all of a sudden you just feel like you should do something; contact that person, email this person or read that book. These are whispers from the universe. It's one thing to see and hear these whispers, but another to act on them. What I've found in my practice and the many I have taught is that once you start living these whispers out and seeing what is on the other side, you come into your authentic self. You start building relationships, standards, boundaries and success so much more strongly. You come into alignment with your path. You find your flow. This is called trusting the universe and it is the key to successfully living intuitively.

Your intuition is usually always there to guide you in the right direction, but sometimes you miss the signs or choose to ignore them. The best way to overcome this is to start noticing when your brain wanders back to a particular thought, and allow it. Slow down and then investigate why you might be feeling this way. Look for patterns, repeated thoughts, and repeated pulls in certain directions. Pay attention to when you feel pulled by something that seems out of the ordinary or surprising. Pay attention to the whispers that seem to ping into being out of nowhere. Remember, intuition does not come from the logical brain. You'll be able to tell if it is your intuition telling you something because you will have the sense that it won't go away; a sensation of knowing you should or should not do something simply keeps mentally tugging at your tail.

INSTINCT VERSUS INTUITION

Instinct and intuition are different. Instinct is an automatic response that has to do with survival. Intuition is more evolved and focused on your highest good and you being your authentic self. One of the biggest signs that intuition is knocking at your door is when you've gone through the decision-making process for something and, while on paper it all seems the right move forward, there is something pulling you back. Instinct says yes. Intuition says no. For example,

---

your instinct may be to stay in your job because it is safe and secure, while your intuition may guide you to leave and start your own business because, deep down, that's the right path for you. Your rational instinct is your ego and will always try to protect you from failure or making a mistake. But by listening to your intuition – your gut feeling – you are guided further than just to survive. Your intuition will help you fight against your fears of failure, so you can make the decision and go for your goals – play big and dream big.

You know your intuition is speaking to you when you feel inspired and excited – like something has lit you up from the inside. This could happen after watching a YouTube video or listening to a podcast or hearing a conversation on the bus. Hearing others' words of wisdom can often help direct your thoughts and spark your intuition so you can begin to follow the path that you are meant to be on. It might feel impulsive or softer in its approach but it will always make your heart sing. Always try to guide with your heart. The more you listen, the happier and more secure you will feel about the choices you make, and the more you can trust your intuition.

DREAM TIME

We all dream. Dreams contain information and, according to many psychologists, they hold knowledge. They provide a window into our mind and into our spirit. They are one of the greatest communication tools our intuition will tap into and utilise because, of course, when we are asleep, the ego is out of the picture. The spirit has complete access to you, without the ego mind rearing its ugly head! When the cognitive mind is busy, it can override the intuitive brain and the subconscious mind, which is the foundation of intuition. When you sleep, your cognitive mind rests and opens space for the subconscious mind to signal you in dreams. Good ones, bad ones – there are often messages in them all. When I have bad dreams, I've found it best to – instead of attaching to them emotionally – view them from the perspective of the information they contain. What is frightening to you? Where are you out of control in life? Is this an opportunity to trust in your spirit and assert your power? Take this opportunity to tune in to your dreams. What could they mean symbolically?

TASK: DREAM JOURNAL

A dream journal is an easy way to record the experiences that you dream about in your sleep. You can start by simply writing down what you remember from your dreams. Don't worry if you find it difficult to recall them, just do it as and when you can. As you continue, you can start to analyse what your dreams mean, especially if you keep having the same kinds of dreams over and over. A dream journal is a type of reflective diary, where you recap on important or unusual things that happen to you. Start by taking a week to write down some of your dreams. Try to interpret them. Allow yourself to become open to receiving and inter-preting these messages for yourself.

Intuition is your master teacher in life.
We learn by reading, hearing, seeing and feeling.
Intuition is another way of knowing.

Your intuition is always there to guide you in the right direction. If sometimes you miss the signs or choose to ignore them, simply trust that there is learning to be felt and allow yourself to find the intention to be open to hear them more clearly the next time. When you live intui-tively, you'll find you live with a feeling that the universe really is meeting you and supporting you with everything you need. You may also find you end up feeling more in your body and this, my friends, is the secret. Listen in to these whispers and act on what you can. When you do, you allow yourself to connect deeply with you and live the life that you were destined to live, not by someone else's compass. Open up to intuition. Expand and explore.

LISTEN TO YOUR BODY

How do you feel in your body? Have you taken time to listen to your body this week, month, year? Being aware of how the universe is engaging with us goes deeper than seeing and acting on the whispers. Your intuition also speaks to you through your body, and the more you cultivate somatic awareness, the more sensitive you become. Intuition allows you to get the first warning signs when anything is off kilter in your body so that you can address it. Think about when you feel stressed or burdened and your shoulders tense up. Or the butterflies in your stomach when you are nervous or excited. That gut feeling or hunch about something that you know just feels right? Hello intuition; it is connecting with you via your body. Now that you have softened into being with your intuition and seeing signs that it might be talking to you, we'll explore how your intuition talks to you through your body.

You know the truth by the way it feels.

Before we go deeper into how your body talks, you must first understand the basics of the human brain. The brain is an incredibly intricate organ that contains about 100 billion neurones and 100 trillion connections.[2] Your brain is command central of all you think, feel and do. It's divided into two halves, or 'hemispheres', and within each half, particular regions control certain functions. As a culture, we have learnt that the body and mind are disconnected. We have also been taught a lot by science about the use of the rational brain; the left side is important for logic and rational thinking. The right side governs abilities that have to do with creativity and the arts.

LEFT SIDE	RIGHT SIDE
Thinking in words	Art awareness
Sequencing	Creativity
Maths and number skills	Imagination
Logic	Intuition
Analytic thought	Insight
Reasoning	Holistic thought
Language	Music awareness

Before making a decision, we might ponder the critical issues, monitor the situation, think rationally with the left side of the brain without considering that the answer might need to come from a place of intuition instead – the right side of the brain. We might use the rational brain when making decisions about anything from crucial business plans or a love interest to what to eat for lunch; for example, 'I ate carbs for breakfast, I should eat protein for lunch.' But what if that gut feeling, that little something instinctual from within, is telling us how we feel beneath those layers of logic? I'm not saying that using the rational part of our brain is redundant and not important because of course it is, but I'm encouraging you to explore your more intuitive side of the brain. In essence, we need to be open to both intuition and reason.

The body is always communicating with us but these signs are often ignored, or we simply cannot feel these symptoms at all because we are living at the speed of light and feel completely disconnected. Many of my clients live in the mind and are completely out of touch with their bodies. I have seen clients with symptoms that have been around for months before they finally seek help in understanding what they mean. Mind and body live in tandem. You can't have one without the other. They are the yin and yang of the human form.

MASCULINE VERSUS FEMININE: THE BASICS

You may have heard of yin and yang? Let's explore what this means in relation to the body, before we go deeper into the idea of listening to our body. If we look back to ancient terms, in both yogic philosophy and traditional Chinese medicine, it's known that we have both a physical body and an energy body called the pranic sheath or *Qi*. The pranic sheath is known to have over 72,000 energy nerves or spiritual currents that are called *Nadis* and each current corresponds to a nerve in the physical body. This is your energy body and in acupuncture they are known as meridians. The word *Nadi* in Sanskrit means 'channel', 'stream' or 'flow'. The *Nadis* channel energy to every single cell in the body but there are points where the *Nadis* accumulate and this is known as a 'chakra' and there are seven key chakras in the body.

There are *Nadis* that govern the feminine and the masculine energies within you. The *Ida Nadi* begins and ends on the left side of the body and is known to control the more feminine aspects of our personalities. It is also the side of the body where we receive. The *Pingala Nadi* begins and ends on the right side of the body and is known to control the more masculine parts of our personalities. From the right side of the body, we give out. The body can show signs of poor-functioning *Ida* and *Pingala Nadis*. For example, signs you have a poor-functioning *Ida Nadi* (feminine energy) can include feeling cold or damp, low mood or depression, low mental energy or sluggish digestion. Signs you may have a poor-functioning

Pingala Nadi (masculine energy) can include feeling hot, angry, having a quick temper, or excessive physical or sexual energy. While yin and yang are not exclusively defined as male and female – and both sexes can be considered either yin or yang within a given context – in terms of their general relation to one another, yin refers to the female and yang to the male. In our bodies, organs can represent either yin or yang.

To live intuitively and to thrive in life we must balance the yin and yang. Although we generally divide humans into female and male, we all share both feminine and masculine qualities and characteristics. When we live intuitively and connect with our higher self, we connect with our internal qualities – both the feminine and masculine characteristics – and, in turn, create a harmonious relationship with ourselves. We need the creativity of the feminine along with the action of the masculine. I see many clients who have lost one part of this balance; living too much in either the feminine or masculine realm.

CASE STUDY: VICKY

Vicky was a writer and film director in London. Her industry was tough and a predominantly masculine domain. She had to be bold and brave, and had spent much of her adult life pouring her energy into her work. Consequently, she lacked a personal and love life. She had been single for ten years and found she was constantly choosing inappropriate men; too young, too busy, or those who were already friends, which only led to blurred lines and boundaries in their relationship.

She embarked on a path of self-discovery and came to me for life coaching. In order to reach the top, Vicky had emulated the masculine way of working. But this wasn't Vicky's natural characteristic, which was causing the confusion and block in calling in a partner. She wasn't attracting men with her authentic self. First, I asked her to be clear on who her ideal partner was; she got specific with what this man looked like physically, how she would feel around him, how he would make her feel. Then I guided her to set boundaries with her friends and around men who just didn't treat her as she wanted to be treated. Finally, I encouraged her to embrace more of her feminine side. Vicky told me that she loved to sing and that it made her feel this soft side of her. I will never forget the sweet sound of her singing in a voice note she sent me. I cried. She had found her feminine force and was able to embrace her two sides, feminine and masculine.

BODY WISE

Now don't get me wrong, I am very pro science and much of my work as a nutritionist is backed by research studies and hard facts. However, on the flipside, there is much that science cannot see and it is here that I will always feel into what signs the body is showing from an energetic point of view. It is here that we can learn what our intuition is telling us.

Start by doing an intuitive body scan. Just as an X-ray machine scans the body in order to gain specific medical details, an intuitive body scan works to provide an energetic portrait. Your physical body has an energy blueprint – the *Nadis* – and so by scanning the body intuitively, you can seek out areas of blocked energy and stress. In my practice, good health is being body aware and able to feel these blockages, and then learning to work on unblocking to allow free-flowing energy and the free functioning of all organs and body systems. Emotional pain can manifest itself in the body as physical pain. Developing intuition means that you can learn to understand your body pain and its message to you. This is developing intuition by using your body to decode your inner condition or your true self. In order to do this you must trust your intuition – trust that your body is a source of this intuition. Using your intuition through listening to your body and its message is a powerful tool for finding health and healing.

Get in touch with your body by sitting somewhere comfortably and taking a quick body scan. Start at the toes; how do they feel? Work your way up to the knees, the hips, the stomach and the chest. How do they feel? The neck, the shoulders, and up to the crown of the head. How do they feel? Look for knots, dark spots, tension, pain or any area that seems to stand out to you during the scan. Note the spot and, if you need to, go back to it for more detail. Do you feel grounded in your legs? Or do they feel heavy? Is there a lightness in any parts of the body? And when you find niggles, are they more of a pain, or an ache? Spend five to ten minutes feeling into your body and, when you're done, write down your findings. Here is what they may mean.

Left side / Feminine side	Symbolises our receptivity as well as the mother, friendships, sisters. Being weak on the left often represents a need to be more bold or assertive.
Right side / Masculine side	Symbolises the father, husband, brothers. Being weak on the right means you perhaps haven't been able to access your own personal power.
Front of the body	Typically represents our immediate situation and the future – usually three to four months in the future. For example, a tightness in the chest can indicate a worry about something coming up in your life.
Back of the body	Represents the past, so perhaps anything you are carrying from the past or thoughts that are based in the past that might be blocking you from moving forwards in life.
Your posture	Says a great deal about you; telling the world about your inner conditions. Do you move easily and flow with energy or do you walk with tension, or bowing down to the ground?

Hands	Represent your productivity or things that you might be holding onto. They also represent how personally powerful we feel. Or are you psychically holding onto something too much? Is it time to let go?
Head	Represents your thought processes and how you conceptualise the world. Are you prone to headaches? Do you feel limited in your resources? Is there some thinking that could be changed?
Neck	Symbolises self-expression and communication. It represents how you communicate with the world. Do you have thyroid problems or neck pain? Are you expressing yourself and being heard enough? Are you speaking your truth? I find in my practice that anyone with a highly functioning thyroid is far too busy; a low-functioning thyroid reveals difficulty with expression or someone who is keeping themselves silent. The neck also represents how we perceive others may be talking about us.
Eyes	Represent how you see things and your ability to view things differently or from a new perspective.
Ears	Can indicate how you may have heard something you didn't want to hear or on the flipside, something you need to listen to more deeply.
Shoulders	Show responsibility; what you put on yourself but also what you are taking on weight-wise. Is this your weight or the weight of someone else?
Chest and heart	Represent emotions and love. Heartache comes when we feel a loss romantically. I find many clients have chest pains or heart conditions after loss.
Lungs	Symbolise our ability to give and receive. Just like the air we breathe in and out, this represents our cycle of life – the flow of life.

Stomach and digestive system	Represent your mental and emotional processes and how you deal with these processes in life and the world. How you process experiences in the world is reflected back in the state of health of your digestive system. Butterflies in the stomach are an emotional experience of the unknown and excitement. If you have a tendency to eat very quickly, what is this saying about how you process information? Are you trying to squash things down without really giving yourself time to work out how you feel?
Reproductive organs and system	Symbolise our sensuality, creative expression and emotions, and how we relate to our body. If you have difficulty in accepting your body it can often result in issues around this part of the body. I see endless clients with hormone imbalances and many of them need support in working with self-love, care and compassion.
Legs	Indicate moving forwards. What are you thinking about your ability to develop and grow – literally moving forwards? How powerful do you think you are in creating the life you want? The legs show our ability to be powerful and navigate the world, accomplishing goals and dreams.
Knees	Indicate self-expression, taking action when thinking about your desires.
Feet	Symbolise our ability to feel grounded, our connections and ability to receive support. When I see issues with the feet I will always ask, do you feel supported right now? Are you comfortable in your own home, at work, in life?
Skin	Symbolises how we feel protected or safe in our environment, or something we feel is not safe for us to express, such as repressed anger or emotions towards a partner, boss or parent.

Be open and willing to hear your body. I'm not talking about every niggle and pain here, but more what you feel with ongoing bodily issues – the recurring ones that could be your intuition showing you something. If you get an uncomfortable physical feeling when you're trying to make a decision, pay attention. Do you feel light or heavy? Have a sick feeling in your gut? Struggle with a headache or diarrhoea? It could just be the result of stress responses activated by false fear, but it could also be your intuition ringing loud and clear.

Your body will express what you need to know. Bodily sensations may come up, so be willing to see them as information. Mind your thoughts so that your body can align itself into the right place with little shifts to health – and by using your intuition.

THE POWER OF TRUST

Humans by nature have a need for fulfilment and more often than not, we look elsewhere for it, instead of tuning in to what makes us feel fulfilled. We are naturally conditioned to seek out a need for approval. We literally grow up with it and get used to it right from the beginning of life. For example, being guided by our parents and having teachers that explain to us how the world works. On certain levels, it's great to have these externals to give us direction but often I find clients become too accustomed to the concept and end up constantly searching for someone to offer approval on what they are doing. Self-approval doesn't seem to be enough. Being able to trust in your choices and be led by intuition is a block I see in many of my clients. I get it; it can be hard to trust in something you can't see. So how do we know what is intuition and what is fear? How do we learn to trust our intuition? This is what we'll explore in this section.

I want you to think about being a child. Do you remember the feelings around believing in the Easter Bunny, Father Christmas and the Tooth Fairy? Although they were unseen and mysterious, you believed in them, right? As you grew older, you worked through the practicalities of Santa getting to every single home in the whole wide world, delivering gifts from his house in the North Pole. You stopped believing. But I want you to think back to when you did believe. How did it feel to believe? This is just like the relationship you have with your intuition. You don't need to see it to believe it. You feel it. It's a deep-rooted inner sense of knowing that you feel. It's yours and no one else's.

FEAR VERSUS INTUITION

The question I get asked the most is: 'How do I know when to trust my intuition and when to disregard it?' Clients have been in situations where they are confused by intuition. They felt like they couldn't decide between two choices. What tends to be happening here is that they aren't experiencing intuition, but fear. Don't use your intuition if you are using your head too much; your ego will be coming through and challenging your intuition. The ego comes through as fear and often gets in the way of trusting our intuition. We have so much chatter in our head and it's just all too noisy. This chatter comes as doubt, worry, judgement and fears about what people think, their perception of us, or that we might not be good enough, smart enough, or doing the right thing. Fear and intuition can easily be confused, mostly because they are both experienced as a gut feeling – and I mean that literally.

So how do we distinguish gut feelings based on fear from gut feelings that signal our intuition? The most important thing that separates fear from intuition is that intuition is only ever about the present. There's no worrying about past or future involved. Just the now. Intuition is also very neutral in feeling. It's unemotional and feels expansive. Fear, however, is highly charged, with emotions and feelings of heaviness. Fear often focuses on the future or past, delving into old psychological wounds. It can feel restrictive. Reliable intuition feels right; it has a compassionate and affirming tone to it, confirms that you are on target, without having an overly positive or negative feeling about it. If you want to distinguish fear from intuition imagine a time in your life when you felt most happy. Notice the feeling in your stomach as you visualise how special you felt, loved, abundant. This will feel expansive. This is intuition. Now think about something that scares you – something destructive, like losing your job or partner. This will feel restrictive or like a shrinking sensation. This is fear.

One of the main ways fear gets in the way of intuition is by keeping you safe. The brain is designed to keep you safe by way of keeping you living in your past experiences. If you had a bad experience in the past – perhaps you were judged because of a choice you made – fear will stop you doing the same thing again. But there is a learning in all of our mistakes and this is very simply our brain (and fear) trying to protect you. Intuition, however, will be the spark that pulls you forward to new experiences. It's the spark of desire, something perhaps a bit radical but that just feels right. It's a bit like love. You may have been hurt before but that can't stop you taking a leap with someone new the next time. All relationships are different, just like all experiences are different. Like my mum used to say, 'When you know, you know.' Stop staying safe.

BOOSTING YOUR TRUST MUSCLE

It's important to put faith in what your body and spirit are trying to tell you. I call this boosting your trust muscle. If you've made decisions based on fear before, you have to get in touch with the part of you that tried to warn you, so that you can trust it the next time. If you want to distinguish fear from intuition, write down everything that you are fearful of. This will allow you to recognise when a gut feeling is based on one of your fears, and by way of brain-dumping – as I've described before – you can see those fears right in front of you; you can face them head-on. When we are fearful we tend to make rash decisions or believe that we are following our intuition because of how strong the mental voice can become. When you are faced with an important decision, try writing down on a piece of paper all your fears surrounding the situation. Making your fears visible will help you to determine whether the voice within you is driven by fear or clear knowing.

What's in the way of you using your intuition?

Are you ready to release your resistance? Don't call yourself crazy when you get an intuitive hunch. Often, the cognitive mind argues with intuition rather than trusting it. By trusting it, you might get yourself into intuitive knowing – into alignment with your path and purpose.

IDENTITY: AN INTUITIVE LIFE

Now you've explored how to connect with your intuition, let's look at how we use it in daily life and how it allows us to find and live our true purpose using the trust we've found. Intuition is a tool, and a tool you can use for life. It's there, always there, inviting you to take it on a journey. If you chose to engage, you will reap wonderful rewards. Intuition functions regardless of the manner in which we utilise it. Living with your intuition can guide you deeply, often in unrecognised ways. Just like regular exercise, the more you use your intuition, the stronger it and you become. The more you use it as a tool to connect to your day-to-day, your mini goals and your WOW goals, the deeper your spiritual growth will thrive and the more connected you will feel to both your body and your higher self. It also strengthens you as you use it.

TASK: LEARNING FROM THE PAST

Much of learning how to engage with intuition as a life tool is understanding when we have and haven't used it in the past. This can help us to be able to watch out for it communicating with us and be able to trust it in the future. Take your journal and find a quiet space to sit and reflect. Recall a negative experience from your past, ideally something fairly recent. This can be an argument, an injury or an event. Allow yourself to think about the hours or moments before this thing happened; think back to whether you got any feelings that urged you to do something different or steer clear? Were you wary of travelling that day or did you already feel a niggle in your shoulder that you went on to injure? Maybe you got a gut feeling something wasn't right. Maybe you had had a strange dream the night before, or perhaps a vision. If so, did you pay attention to that feeling, dream or vision, or did you talk yourself out of it? Try to remember exactly how you felt that day and write down as many details as possible.

You might have a few experiences like this so write them down too. I remember when I started my company Rooted Living, I asked a friend to team up with me on the supper clubs and catering side of the business; we – in my eyes – were the dream team. One night I had a strange dream and when I woke up I said to my boyfriend, 'She doesn't want to be part of the business, I'm going to do it alone.' Lo and behold that very morning I got a text saying that she would like to meet. I just knew that she wasn't feeling it the way I was. I felt that my intuition had come to me in the night.

Now don't get me wrong, I'm all for living in the moment, but for every day I let life lead the way, there is a day that I get clear on what I want. If you want to trust in your intuition, you have to trust in what you want in life. You have to get clear on your goals so you can trust that your intuition will guide you to the right destination. Ask yourself each day: What feeds my soul? What feels good? And then allow yourself to sit with that question. The answers will come. If it feels good, use your journal. Once you get clear on what you want in life, make an action plan. The brain loves a plan. Once you turn down the volume on fear and worry, you can turn up the volume of a can-do, high-achieving attitude (more on this in Week 5). You can turn up the volume on your authenticity and intuitive living.

Learning to live intuitively doesn't come overnight. It's a process. If you're putting a lot of pressure on yourself, take a load off. The pressure of having to make a quick decision tends to inhibit the flow of intuition. While intuition can work under stressful circumstances, if you have the option to slow down, take it. Putting decisions on the back burner can help you to relax and adopt a new perspective. From here you'll be open and more easily guided by the presence of your intuitive knowing. If you are faced with a situation where you are unsure whether fear or intuition is calling the shots, come up with a range of solutions and really think about each scenario. Take time to visualise each choice as clearly as you can and then pay attention to how each option feels. Whichever option feels the most right is the choice you need to go for.

If life gets sticky and you need guidance from your intuition, don't be afraid to ask for help; ask and you will receive! The universe will deliver. Sometimes you might get from A to B on a straight road, and sometimes you'll go around the houses, but intuition will guide you to the right decision. Put it out to the universe – what do you need help with? Seek things out. Nothing is too small or too large; it's just a case of asking.

If something is blocked, ask why?

TASK: ASKING FOR HELP

Grab your journal and ask yourself the following questions. Write down what comes up.

1.   How easy or hard is it for you to ask for help? Why?
2.   What are your beliefs about asking for or receiving help?
3.   Your intuition improves when you ask. Right now, close your eyes and enquire within. What do you need to do to get more clarity, confidence and consistency with your intuition? How are you holding yourself back?
4.   If you are standing in your own way, enquire now as to what you can do to let go and move on.

The answers are there. Note down how intuition could help you in health, your job, your money mindset, family or love life. Can you believe that you have great health, wealth, a wonderful family, enough money? When you believe in your intuition making this happen, how does it feel?

Intuition exists in fullness all the time, but it's up to you to connect with it and use it. A strong intuitive connection offers tremendous benefits. Following intuition inspires us to dream big, guides us to manifest our desires, enlivens us to the richness of everyday moments, and works to enhance life on every level.

INTUITION: THE TOOLKIT

How are you feeling about using your intuition now? For many of you, it seems fairly straightforward and you feel like you are tapping into it already. For others, the inner critic might still be calling the shots and you may be finding it hard to hear it. Remember that wherever you are, it's okay. Using intuition doesn't happen overnight and it's a lifelong development. To round up this week, here are some additional tools to focus on to connect further to your intuition. Try using one each day and mix them up. Remember, sometimes it is the things you resist the most that you need the most.

BRAIN-DUMP: MORNING PAGES

For this section I want you to take your journal and, each morning for a week, spend five minutes writing the first things that come into your head. This can be anything from a to-do list, last night's dream, a feeling or something more profound. The choice is yours! Morning pages teach you not to judge your mood and not to judge yourself. When you write freely, you can find yourself freer in your life. You allow yourself to hear when the universe is responding to you. You may write down ways in which you have heard your intuition telling you the next step. These morning pages allow you to see the picture clearly. It might not always be what you want to see but, through this practice, you can learn that a negative morning page may have the outcome of a great day. It teaches you that emotions and feelings are transient. Allow five minutes or two to three pages minimum. Show no one and then get on with your day.

CULTIVATE A HEALTHY PINEAL GLAND

The pineal gland is a tiny, pea-sized gland shaped like a pine cone that resides in the centre of the brain. It's known to hold the secrets to spiritual wisdom, inspiration and psychic awareness and is vital for physical, mental and spiritual health, while also being a gateway to higher consciousness. Traditionally, the pineal gland is said to be the third-eye chakra, otherwise known as Ajna or the eyebrow chakra, which is set back and between the eyes. The pineal gland produces melatonin and regulates our daily and seasonal circadian rhythms. Melatonin is the chemical in charge of our sleep cycles and the quality of our sleep, and it also regulates the onset of puberty. Serotonin, the neurotransmitter or happy chemical responsible for our mood, is transformed into melatonin only in the pineal gland. Our pineal gland can get blocked through poor diet, exposure to toxins in the environment and the food we eat, stress and modern life, and eventually it hardens, calcifies and can shut down. Gasp. Take time to nurture your pineal gland through meditation by focusing on this point. You can also reduce your fluoride intake.

PRACTISING AFFIRMATIONS

Every day, come up with a sentence that you truly want to remind yourself of or that you want to experience on that day. What do you desire? What do you want? This will change the way you feel. You'll start to feel empowered by the life that you are creating. No need to process these affirmations, just observe and allow them to sink into your mind and body. This allows you to talk to yourself in a very affirmative way too. Each must be heart-centred and, as you say it, think about how it feels. Speak the affirmation to yourself. The more you talk about these things, and communicate to yourself, the more you will be connected to your intuition and thus be stronger in your life. When you become so comfortable with yourself, you are empowering yourself. This really is about practice – what you put in, you get out.

ESCAPE FROM ROUTINE

With our rules and our fast, hectic lifestyles, we often get so busy in our routines that we forget to try something new. Get away. Slow down. Go on a retreat, take a sabbatical, or just spend a day in new surroundings with nothing planned. If time is not a constraint, you can take the scenic route home, or get off public transport a stop early to walk a new way home. Practise spontaneity by doing something out of the ordinary. Write a kind note to your housemate or loved one. Take out some paper and write whatever is inspiring you, even if you are in a setting where you normally wouldn't do it. Leave an inspiring quote on the fridge at work. Try something new. Look up! How often do we see only the things in our immediate eye line? What would happen if you looked up once in a while? When you're overly busy, it's hard to be sensitive to the quiet voice of intuition. Try clearing your schedule and see if your intuition pipes up.

CHAKRA MEDITATION:
SEARCHING FOR BLOCKAGES

Similar to a body scan, this meditation searches for blockages within the body. When your chakras are healthy and clear, your life can flow smoothly. When they are sluggish, shut down or weak, the imbalance can show up as a physical symptom affecting that particular area of your body. Chakras are centres of energy found in everyone, and these centres receive, transform and distribute that energy throughout the body. Chakras play an important part in our physical, emotional and spiritual health and, thus, our ability to live intuitively. If you are experiencing a physical or emotional imbalance, this meditation will rebalance and stimulate the energy flow of your chakras. The result is feeling more confident, energised and at peace.

Start by sitting or lying down comfortably. Close your eyes and come into your body. Take a deep breath and feel the way it flows through your body. Take a body scan and breathe into areas of tightness, aches or pains. Bring your awareness into the chakras, starting from the root chakra up to the crown chakra. Below is a list of the chakras, their colours, meaning and the mantra associated with each. For each chakra, direct your inner visualisation to this point on the body. Tap into how it feels. Imagine the colour of the chakra radiating through your body and repeat the mantra ten times, before moving up to the next chakra. Take your time with this practice.

Root chakra (Muladhara)
Colour: Red
Mantra: Lam
Location: Base of spine
Meaning: Governs your connection to the world, your fundamental
needs such as food and shelter but also how you feel grounded
emotionally

Sacral chakra (Svadhisthana)
Colour: Orange
Mantra: Vam
Location: Below the navel
Meaning: Your creative process; it governs both your sexuality,
reproductive organs and imagination. It is essential for coping
with new experiences and exploration

Solar plexus chakra (Manipura)

Colour: Yellow

Mantra: Ram

Location: Above the navel, in the stomach

Meaning: Your digestion as well as how you psychically digest
things – how you embrace experience

Heart chakra (Anahata)

Colour: Green

Mantra: Yam

Location: Heart

Meaning: How you form emotional connections to others

Throat chakra (Vishuddha)

Colour: Blue

Mantra: Ham

Location: Throat

Meaning: Self-expression and communication

Third-eye chakra (Ajna)

Colour: Indigo

Mantra: Sham

Location: In between the eyebrows

Meaning: How you see the world, your insight and intuition

Crown chakra (Sahasrara)

Colour: Purple

Mantra: Om

Location: Top of the head

Meaning: Sense of peace, wellbeing and confidence

Feed Your Soul

The Diet Dilemma
No Fads, Just Feeding
The Hunger Scale
Introducing Intuitive Eating
Dealing with Feelings: Emotional Eating
Dealing with Friends: Social Occasions
Feed Your Soul: The Toolkit

THE DIET DILEMMA

Women are all shapes and sizes. Some are tall, some are short. Some have big boobs, some have small boobs. Some are able to eat and eat without gaining a single pound. Others find they can't even look at a piece of chocolate without gaining weight. But what do many of us have in common? We are all encouraged or have a desire to be smaller or change our bodies, that's what. Let me start by asking you, have you ever been on a diet? Have you tried the latest fad food craze? Or perhaps you are currently on a diet? You may be someone who has been on a diet all of your life? Welcome to Week 4, where I'll be explaining all things food; exploring fad diets, what dieting does to the body and why diet culture is dead. Welcome to the concept of Intuitive Eating – I'm hopeful that this book is about to change your life forever.

There is always a new diet to try – one that promises that you'll live your best life or gain health and happiness, if only you would lose those pounds! Dr Atkins takes away whole food groups, the 5:2 promotes complete deprivation for two days of the week, or then there's the Zone diet, which is possibly the most confusing diet ever known. Who has time to measure every grain and count every calorie? As Susie Orbach explains in her book *Fat Is a Feminist Issue*, 'diets turn normal eaters into people who are afraid of food'. Food has become the enemy and turned us into compulsive, controlling and confused beings who are now completely lost when it comes to knowing how to eat. ENOUGH. It's time to embrace our bodies as they are, and reject the obsession to be thin based on someone else's ideal of what it is to be beautiful or healthy.

So what is a diet mentality? Remember how, in Week 2, I explained about imprints and the stories you've absorbed? Well, it's these that create the diet mentalities; ideas of how you should eat in order to be 'healthy'. A diet mentality can be hard to recognise. Whereas a diet is a meal plan or a set of rules – something that dictates what, when and how much you eat – a diet mentality may be lurking in the shadows. It's a way of filtering your food choices, often without you even realising it. Treating you like a puppet on a string, a diet keeps you hanging without a sense of security and control. A diet mentality is different: it's certain rules you cling onto because you don't want to 'diet', but you want your body to look and feel a certain way. With a diet mentality, the inner monologue around food choices might read something like this:

- If I eat carbs, I'll get fat.
- If I exercised more, I'd be happier/get the man of my dreams/a better job.
- To be healthy is to put my body through restriction.
- To control my weight, I have to control my calories.
- I shouldn't eat that, it's bad for me.
- I should look like (insert Kim K, Gisele, etc.) to be valued.
- My body is not good enough.
- I shouldn't eat after 6pm.
- I've had carbs for lunch, I won't have carbs for dinner.

- I only eat carbs before a run.
- I don't eat 'processed' food.
- I shouldn't snack.

Do any of these statements resonate with you? When you feel hungry, a diet mentality may ask things like:

- When was the last time I ate?
- I've just had breakfast, why am I still hungry?
- How many calories does this have in it and will this be over my quota for the day?

A diet mentality gives you absolutely no wiggle room in your food consumption. You're always in the balancing act of eating what you want and eating what you think you 'should' eat. It decides your food choices for you, not taking into consideration your cravings that day and other very important factors, such as your mood, how much sleep you've had or, quite simply, how hungry you are from day to day. A diet mentality constantly bombards you with rules and over time will completely block your body from telling you what it needs to be nourished and to thrive. It's the antithesis of intuitive eating. A huge factor in overcoming a diet mentality is understanding what dieting does to the body. This is no scaremongering; this is truth – from studies to my clinic, I have seen it all. As far as the body is concerned, dieting – certainly extreme dieting – is a form of starvation.

- Chronic dieting teaches the body to retain more fat when you start eating again. This is something I personally found after years of starvation followed by bingeing. Low-calorie diets double the enzymes that make and store fat in the body. This is basically done as a tool for the body to store more energy – for survival. That's what our body does for us – it enables us to survive.[1]

- Chronic dieting slows the rate of weight loss with each attempt to diet. This has been shown in human and rat studies.[2]
- It can decrease metabolism by triggering the body to become more efficient at utilising calories by lowering the body's need for energy.[3]
- It can increase binges and cravings. Both humans and rats have been shown to overeat after food restriction. It stimulates the brain to launch a cascade of cravings and eat more. After substantial weight loss, rats have been shown to prefer eating more fat.[4]

THE VICIOUS DIET CYCLE

Many of you will have found yourself in 'the diet dilemma', jumping off and on the diet bandwagon over and over. The hopelessness of dieting is best explained in the Dieter's Dilemma chart created by psychologists John P. Foreyt and G. Ken Goodrick in their book, *Living without Dieting*. The dieter's dilemma is triggered by the desire to be thin, which leads to dieting, which is where the dilemma unfolds. Dieting increases the urge to eat and crave foods, so the dieter goes into overdrive and overeats. The cycle starts again, often with the dieter at a heavier weight than when they started! I always found this chart incredibly helpful both personally and in my clinic. I welcome you to draw this out for yourself and stick it on the fridge door as a gentle reminder to NOT diet.

Diet culture stands in the way of you living authentically and intuitively. It convinces you that certain bodies have more value than others and instils the notion of fat phobia, which in our culture is big business. If we all continued to feel bad about our bodies and feared being larger than the supposed perfect weight or body shape, then we'd spend any amount of money on products, meal plans and quick-fix exercise programmes to try to remedy the situation. If we believe diet culture's stories, then it wins and we lose. But if you can recognise these diet mentalities and stories for what they are, you can also understand that you have the power to let them go. So, are you ready to overcome your diet mentalities?

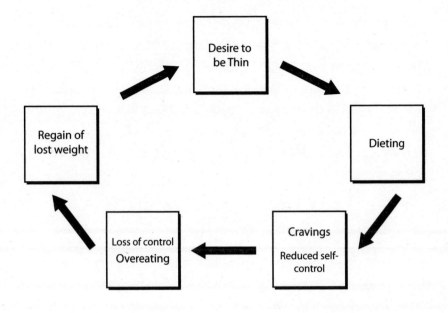

TASK: IDENTIFY YOUR DILEMMA

Grab your journal and find a quiet space, both externally and within. Take yourself back to when you first thought food was an enemy or something to be scared of. Where did this come from? From whom or what was it created? Then take yourself on a journey through your childhood to now: what mentalities have been imprinted on you about what you should and shouldn't eat? Here are some pointers that may help you:

- How did you eat as a child?
- What rules did your mother and father eat with?
- What comparisons have you made around food growing up?
- What stories have you heard about dieting from the media or people that you've taken on as your own?
- What food rules do you live by or think from time to time – such as carbs are bad, sugar is bad or when food should be eaten?

Write down all of your diet mentalities and then reread them to yourself. Think about when you use them – is it daily or just now and again? Write it down next to each one. Start to connect with your diet mentalities. The quicker you can accept them, the quicker you can change them. You have the power to set down diet culture's stories and write new ones of your own. You have the power to unlearn them. It's time to create your own. Are you ready to banish fads? Let's look at how in the next section.

NO FADS, JUST FEEDING

There's a societal pressure to be slim, driven by a cultural obsession. We've become so dissatisfied with our bodies that we've become afraid of them, and even more afraid of what we eat. Meanwhile, people only blame themselves; they feel that a lack of willpower, no self-control or bad genetics are the reasons they can't lose weight, which ultimately sends them even further down the dieting hole. It's a vicious cycle. To help pinpoint and overcome your personal dieting trap, you must first identify with the type of dieter you are and your triggers.

TYPES OF DIETERS

In their book *Intuitive Eating*, originally published in 1995, registered dieticians Evelyn Tribole and Elyse Resch identify eight types of dieters:

#1

Eating style: Careful Eater

Trigger: Fitness and health

Characteristic: Appears to be the perfect eater; anguishes over each food morsel and its effect on the body. On the surface, this person seems health- and fitness-oriented.

#2

Eating style: Unconscious Eater
Trigger: Eating while doing something else at the same time
Characteristic: This person is often unaware that he/she is eating, or how much is being eaten. To sit down and simply eat is often viewed as a waste of time. Eating is usually paired with another activity to be productive. There are many subtypes.

#2.1

Eating style: Chaotic Unconscious Eater
Trigger: Overscheduled life
Characteristic: This person's eating style is haphazard – gulp 'n' go when the food is available. Seems to thrive on tension.

#2.2

Eating style: Refuse-not Unconscious Eater
Trigger: Presence of food
Characteristic: This person is especially vulnerable to candy jars, or food present in meetings or sitting openly on the kitchen counter.

#2.3

Eating style: Waste-not Unconscious Eater
Trigger: Free food
Characteristic: This person's eating drive is often influenced by the value of the food dollar and is susceptible to all-you-can-eat buffets and free food.

#2.4

Eating style: Emotional Unconscious Eater
Trigger: Uncomfortable emotions
Characteristic: Stress or uncomfortable feelings trigger eating – especially when alone.

#3

Eating style: Professional Dieter

Trigger: Feeling fat

Characteristic: This person is perpetually dieting, often trying the
latest commercial diet or diet book.

#4

Eating style: Intuitive Eater

Trigger: Biological hunger

Characteristic: This person makes food choices without experiencing
guilt or an ethical dilemma. Honours hunger, respects fullness,
enjoys the pleasure of eating.

What I've found most important – and the key to a sustainable weight
and positive body image – is an understanding of your personal eating
habits. Once you identify your habits, you can take the steps to maintain
the healthy ones and change the ones that are, quite literally, weighing
you down. Personally, I've found there to be four key types of dieters.
Below I outline each identity and the first step to overcome this mentality.

THE EMOTIONAL EATER

The Emotional Eater celebrates with food and commiserates with food.
They use food as a crutch to give them support when they are stressed or
upset. They are usually unable to distinguish between types of emotions
that they feel and have an inability to stop using food as a coping mechanism. The food doesn't often solve the problem and, thus, they end up
in a worse state given that the guilt associated with eating the food only
creates yet another problem.

First steps . . .

Getting to grips with emotions is key for the Emotional Eater. If this is
you, start by checking in with how you're feeling throughout the day. If

you're feeling emotional, think about what you can do to make yourself feel better, without food. Create a list of 'non-food' ways to make yourself feel better; to celebrate or elevate your mood. Do you need a chat with a friend, a manicure or a massage? If you're stressed, would some deep breathing help, or taking a walk in your lunch break for some fresh air?

THE HABITUAL EATER

The Habitual Eater is very rigid with their food consumption. They live and eat according to sheer habit – same foods, same time, every week. For the Habitual Eater it's often difficult for them to acknowledge when they are hungry or not, because they eat so rigidly each day. Even if they aren't hungry at dinner, they'll eat because it's 'dinner time' and that's what they habitually think they should do. They love routine and hate random or spontaneous events, such as a late-night dinner. If they are eating out, they have a tendency to want to know the menu before they've even stepped foot in the restaurant. They often use calorie-counting apps.

First steps . . .
The key to overcoming this diet mentality is to bring some spontaneity into the kitchen. Perhaps take up a cooking course or try a new recipe from a different cookbook each week. Afraid of stepping out of their comfort zone, the Habitual Eater has to expand and explore at their own pace. If you resonate with this and you use calorie-counting apps, turn them off immediately. Allow yourself – for one week – complete permission to eat whatever you want. If need be, it can help to find a ritual elsewhere, such as a morning meditation practice, journalling or walking to work. Maybe, just maybe, learn to take a walk on the wild side of the kitchen.

THE INDULGENT EATER

The Indulgent Eater cannot say no to food. Cake at the office, advertisements on the bus, samples handed out at the supermarket – they are a sucker for a free bite. The Indulgent Eater overeats, not from hunger, but from external cues. They'll always have dessert because they are eating out for dinner and feel like they should indulge. They often find themselves feeling guilty for eating something they weren't hungry for and, thus, end up trying to balance out their food intake with skipping meals.

First steps . . .

Shaking off the 'I see therefore I eat' mentality is key for the Indulgent Eater, along with tapping into and honouring your hunger. Start by writing down what your external cues are, whether that's always having choc-olate to hand at the office or going out to dinner a lot. Before allowing yourself to overindulge, ask yourself, 'Am I hungry?' and 'Do I really want this?' This can help you tap into your body's hunger. If your stomach says no but your head says yes, honour your stomach and save some room for when you are hungry.

THE ALL-OR-NOTHING EATER

The All-or-Nothing Eater is either on or off the diet rails. This eater is fairly knowledgeable about what basic health is and has a good understanding of nutrition, but finds it hard to find balance with their food consumption. They see food as 'good' or 'bad', and very often start the day 'good', with green smoothies and juices, but by 4pm have devoured an entire pizza and box of chocolates. Their constant restriction (on) always creates a need for overindulgence (off) and means they often feel guilty, which only makes matters worse.

First steps . . .

For the All-or-Nothing Eater, giving themselves permission is key. If this is you, take your foot off the food pedal and feel into your food choices. Write down those foods you label as 'good' and 'bad' and try to ease up on these rigid food rules. Try to identify how self-destructive your mentality is and support yourself in knowing that no food is bad, or good. Trust that your food intake will balance itself and that one 'bad' food choice doesn't ruin your entire day.

DITCHING THE DIET MENTALITY

The first step in breaking any diet mentality is to make the decision to stop dieting. I know, your palms are probably sweating just thinking about it. But I promise you, everything is going to be okay! I want you to become the person who gives you permission to let go of all the stories that you inherited about food, body size and health, and all of the mentalities that you live by. To drop the pursuit of weight loss and the obsessive thoughts and behaviours around food, you need to stop believing the stories that diet culture has told you. Not only are those stories false, but they are holding you back from being who you really are in the body that you own. Imagine what you could do if you let go of these mentalities that take up so much of your mental space. What would you dream up if you weren't constantly thinking about what to eat and how to change your body? Imagine what it would be like to have the time to devote to interests and pursuits other than food, fitness and health. What have you always wanted to try, but were putting off until you changed your body? Imagine what it would be like to take pleasure in food and movement. If you didn't feel like you had to police and monitor yourself in all these arenas, how much more could you enjoy your life?

JOURNALLING: FOOD DIARY

Get to know your food habits by journalling and keeping an eye on your narrative. Please start writing down everything that you eat, at what times and how these meals make you feel. Then go deeper. Here are a few questions you could use as a guide:

- How did you feel before, during and after eating?
- Are there any noticeable repeated thoughts and ideas that go through your head when you choose and eat foods?
- Are there any emotions that come up when you eat?
- Are there any physical symptoms?

This exercise is not about eating perfectly or a way to control your consumption (do not eat what you think you should eat throughout the day just for the diary), this is about exploring you and your eating habits. It helps you become aware of feelings, thoughts, patterns, habits, behaviours, reactions and physical symptoms that you may not have paid much attention to before. There is no right or wrong in this exercise. Just enquire and speak to your body. Do not try to do this because you think you 'should'. Do not try to get answers or even understand. Just do it. Answers and insights will come when it's the right time.

THE HUNGER SCALE

Eat when you're hungry. Don't eat when you're not. Seems like a simple idea, right? Hunger is a natural and necessary urge but sadly much of our society is being sold the idea of suppressing or ignoring hunger every day. From the diet industry, well-meaning friends or family members to celebrity culture (cue Kim Kardashian promoting a hunger-suppressing lollipop!), we are being encouraged to ignore our hunger. In this section we start to build on the knowledge of anti-diets and how we understand and honour hunger, plus what happens when we don't. Here are some examples you may have heard:

- Drink a glass of water before eating a meal and you will eat less.
- Avoid snacking to lose weight.
- You have 35 points a day and once you use them up, eat celery or zero-points foods.

- Skinny tea helps to suppress your appetite.
- Don't eat after 6pm to lose weight.

These are diet mentalities just like I've established in the last section, and they take you further away from understanding and honouring your hunger. To understand how to find a balance with our hunger, we must first look at why we may over- and undereat to begin with and how to overcome it.

YOUR BODY IS CONFUSED

Today's world is a busy place; we lead hectic lives. Many of you may rush out the door and grab whatever's convenient for breakfast, or maybe you don't eat anything at all. Your day consists of meetings or errands so you eat lunch on the go or quickly at your desk. At night, after a long day you come home exhausted and eat something easy and quick, maybe even a takeaway or ready meal you've picked up en route. You'll eat it on the sofa or the night bus home. Of course, this may be an exaggeration and your day isn't always like this, but how often are you skipping meals, eating on the go, or eating while checked out? How does your body know it's time to eat? Without the correct signals, your body will not turn on the necessary digestive functions to digest your meal and assimilate the nutrients you're taking in. When you do actually eat, your body will take longer to relay the neurotransmitter signals that tell your brain you've had enough, meaning you'll consume more food than your body actually needs. For many of you, this way of eating brings little satisfaction, so you end up raiding the fridge for seconds moments later.

YOU'RE MEASURING FOOD IN THE WRONG WAY

Diet rules and so-called experts have convinced you that you should be measuring your meals in ways that completely distance you from having a real connection to your food and your hunger. Hands up who has used a Fitbit, food trackers or calorie counters? Me included, my arms raised high; I've used them all. I'm not saying these devices aren't useful, because they are. I loved getting into running with the Nike app because it kept me going knowing the distances I covered each week got longer. But when it comes to hunger, every day is going to be different. Sometimes you'll need two breakfasts, and others none at all. Measurements can be important, but if you're working on honouring your hunger, know that it will change daily. It is time to measure your food based on how you're feeling.

ARE YOU REALLY HUNGRY FOR FOOD?

Stressed, bored, confused or fatigued – your body isn't actually craving nutrients or calories; it's craving comfort. Perhaps you are having a stressful day, or you're in the middle of a major life transition, or maybe you are just really exhausted from a few bad nights' sleep. Food can be a great symbolic substitute but your body is reacting to it like it's a drug; literally changing your biochemical reactions. If you're out of control with how you eat due to your outside environment, it's time to explore the situations that surround your overeating experiences. It's okay to let yourself receive comfort in this way from time to time, but relying on food to regulate your mood is a dangerous habit, creating a vicious cycle of depending on food to calm you followed by an even higher stress response as you feel shame and guilt for overeating. It's time to find another coping mechanism.

So as you can see, there is a lot that can take you away from your hunger. While many of you will probably consider overeating in particular to be a willpower problem, I promise you it's not. Connecting your mind and body allows you to tap into how you are feeding yourself in all areas of your life. By being more conscious of your eating patterns, staying present at your chosen mealtimes and honouring your hunger, especially during times of stress or discomfort, you can find new ways to grow and even newer ways to feel more nourished.

TASK: THE HUNGER SCAN

This simple body scan can be great to understand where and why you are hungry. Becoming aware of how your surroundings affect you as well as your physical and emotional hunger can allow you to feed yourself in the best way possible.

Start by finding somewhere comfortable and taking three deep, long breaths, in through the nose and out through the mouth. How does your body feel? Nice, uncomfortable or neutral? How is your mood? Are you snappish, grumpy or light and cheery? What does this say about your hunger?

How are your energy levels? Low, high or somewhere in between? Are you sleepy, or vibrant with energy? What could this say about your hunger?

Turn your attention to your body and scan through: How is your head? Achy, dizzy, faint? Or sharp and full of concentration? Your stomach? Empty, growling or yearning? Or too full and heavy? Notice any sensations in the body that might clue you into hunger.

Take three more deep breaths and write down anything that came up.

USING THE HUNGER SCALE

I've worked with clients at both ends of the spectrum and everything in between. Some can't remember the last time they felt hungry, the result of a lifetime using the fear of scarcity to drive their eating patterns. Others push themselves to a point of ravenousness, constantly living with niggles and pains in the body as they ignore the signs that their body needs feeding. Many of my clients go between the two – restricting to a point of pain and then overeating to a different place of pain. Caught

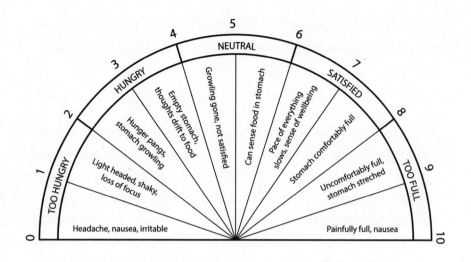

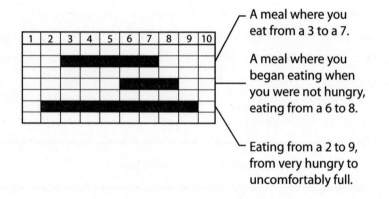

A meal where you eat from a 3 to a 7.

A meal where you began eating when you were not hungry, eating from a 6 to 8.

Eating from a 2 to 9, from very hungry to uncomfortably full.

in the hunger yo-yo, they are lost as to what hunger really feels like. The hunger–fullness scale is a tool used by intuitive-eating specialists worldwide and even our own NHS to help you learn how to tune in to what your body needs and begin to eat more intuitively.

Ideally, a 3–4 is a great place to enjoy a meal. Waiting until you are a 1–2 puts you in danger of overeating. Eating when you are neutral, around 5, might be necessary but isn't the ideal hunger spot for a large meal. And once you begin to feel a fullness, at 6–7, you can start tuning in to how full you want to be. I find many clients look at the hunger scale and realise they are only eating out of boredom, so they don't eat at all. They wait until they are hungry. The process of using the hunger scale is a great start to tuning in to your body and its subtle cues of hunger. If you're someone who thinks that by allowing yourself whatever you want to eat, you'd eat the house down, this will help you manage your hunger; your *actual* hunger. Once you reach the moment of excessive hunger, all intentions of moderate, conscious eating are thrown out of the window. Learning to honour your biological signal sets the stage for rebuilding trust with yourself and food.

Some of you may thrive on breakfast. Or you might find it makes you feel heavy and lethargic before you've even left the house. Some of you need a regular mealtime rather than giving your body mixed signals, so you may need to train your body to know when to expect food. Some people naturally have more energy early in the day, and are therefore better able to digest and metabolise a larger calorie intake; however, others prefer a larger meal later in the day. Experiment. Perhaps try eating a more substantial, protein-rich breakfast one day, with a grain-based meal the next. Play around with the amount of food you are eating at lunch and dinner, and make sure you aren't going too low in the hunger scale before any mealtime, which will create a natural desire to overeat. There's a sweet spot between mild and ravenous hunger, so start to observe when this happens for you. Use your food diary to write down anything you notice.

If you find yourself overeating, observe what it is you are actually eating. Are you physically or emotionally hungry? If you are consuming a tray of chocolates or cookies, are you enjoying the fifth, sixth one or were you satisfied from the first but are now overeating out of an emotional prompt? Our bodies need essential fats, complex carbohydrates, proteins and amino acids. When the body receives these nutrients, it more readily signals the brain that you're satisfied, and full. If the food you consume is deficient in these nutrients, you may continue to crave and eat because your brain–belly connection is broken. It's been shown that it's the micro-nutrient density of a diet that influences the experience of hunger. A high nutrient-density diet provides benefits for long-term health as well as weight-loss stability longer term.[5] Observe why you are eating these foods. Are you hungry? Is it this food that you really need? Allow yourself to observe but, most importantly, without judgement.

If it's measurements that you find tricky, start by using the hunger scale to notice sensations of fullness. It takes 20 minutes for the stomach to message the brain that it's full so if you're eating quickly, you'll miss these signals. Also, think about the quality of your food choices. Even if you eat the exact same things but consume a higher-quality version (like organic, local or homemade), your body may digest it in a more optimal way. You may just feel more satisfied.

Here are some other ways to tune in to your hunger:

VITAMIN A: AWARENESS

Learning to honour your hunger means exploring vitamin A: awareness of what's going on in your life. Start with the simple act of noticing what is happening in your life when you under- or overeat. Look for patterns, similarities, times of day – anything that may be causing this disordered eating. Over time you might just find that a pattern emerges that will allow you to find a softer way to control what's going on that doesn't revolve around food. If it's stress that's causing you to eat more or less, try to make a list of non-food, nourishing activities that can manage this stress response and explore ways to include them in your day, especially during challenging or trying times. Maybe you find taking a short walk on your lunch break, deep breathing, listening to music or getting a weekly massage helps. Any of these activities can short-circuit the desire to overeat as a form of medication. It will take time and practice, but commit to trying this out for a few weeks and notice what happens.

VITAMIN P: PLEASURE

Before and as you eat, allow your body to really take in the scents and look of your meal. Consider choosing food based on the aroma and taste, as well as how it looks and how you think it will feel in the body. This will help to activate your parasympathetic response and start your digestive function before you even begin eating. Think about a time when your house smelled of a home-cooked meal being prepared and how perhaps the aromas triggered your belly to rumble and your mouth to water. An early memory of mine was my mum's rice pudding every weekend, or even the smell of toast coming from the kitchen in the mornings. Start to embrace the need for pleasure from the foods you eat; we are wired to have a pleasurable response to food before it's even consumed. Find pleasure from food and you might just feel more satisfied.

MY THEORY ON THE 4PM SLUMP

I can't tell you how many clients I have had who find the 4pm slump their battleground for overeating. Part of them feels like they need a lift so they eat something sugary to give them a boost, only to feel the slump after their sugar high two to three hours later. It's a vicious cycle. I've found with many women that, once they start a food diary, it becomes clear very quickly that the 4pm slump is not a need for food at all, but instead the time of day when they become tired, grumpy or stressed. It's that time – especially if you've not taken a proper lunch break – when the busyness of the day catches up with you. Instead of reaching for the snacks, try to take a solid hour's lunch break, get some fresh air and make sure to take smaller, five-minute breaks throughout the day, especially if you work at a screen.

INTRODUCING INTUITIVE EATING

Well done, you've made it this far. You've identified many of your diet mentalities and body blocks as well as how to connect to your intuition and honour your hunger. Now let me introduce you to Intuitive Eating – a concept that might just change your life forever. Evelyn Tribole and Elyse Resch introduced the concept in their 1995 book of the same name; they called their approach a '180-degree departure from dieting'. As dieticians they had many clients coming to see them with a desire to lose weight, or with conditions where weight loss would be key to their treatment. Their diet plans would work but, over time, clients would regain the weight and be back at square one. This cycle reinforced negative, self-critical notions that their patients had about themselves – no self-control or an inability to stick to their food plans – turning to guilt. They explored the possibility of devising a new foundation of nutrition that bridged a gap between anti-diet and health. Intuitive Eating was born and, since, there have been over 60 studies to show that it works.[6] Instead of a strong focus on weight loss, deprivation, cutting or counting calories or completely writing off certain foods or food groups, Intuitive Eating teaches you how to eat in a way that supports a kinder and thus healthier relationship with food. The goal is to see health from 360 degrees – meaning on every level, physically, emotionally and mentally.

I first came across Intuitive Eating during my studies as a nutritionist. Alongside my studies, I was working as a PR for many health and well-being companies and so I knew that the media loved a fad; it was part of my job to come up with a way to spin a product to make it newsworthy. I found that while the study of nutrition was incredibly interesting, a lot of the information contradicted itself. Having studied yoga, visualisation tools and meditation, I was already aware of how powerful the mind was for health and, from a personal perspective, how body positivity and self-love were the foundation of my own healing. As with all things, the

Intuitive Eating book fell into my lap, and I quickly fell in love with it. Here, I thought, is something I can work with. It tied everything I knew about dealing with disordered eating from a personal journey with everything I had been learning and questioning about nutrition. Now don't get me wrong, I am still today in awe of and empowered by the effect food can have on the body, and I continue to work as a nutritionist to help those who have conditions ranging from hormone imbalance to skin disorders, BUT when it comes to weight loss, I know a diet just doesn't work. When it comes to disordered eating in any form, a focus on weight loss is absolutely not suitable. I've combined some of the principles of Intuitive Eating with my own toolkit, rich from practices I myself have experienced, plus the skills I have learnt as a life coach to create my programmes and the principles of my business, Rooted Living.

THE PRINCIPLES OF INTUITIVE EATING

Below are the original ten principles of Intuitive Eating as outlined in the book, with my own description of how each works and how it has worked for some of my clients. Some we've touched on before in much greater detail and with my own spin. Others are new but are easily explained and will make sense to you in the greater scheme of everything you've learnt already.

REJECT THE DIET MENTALITY

We've worked though the idea of this one already. Reminder: if dieting is the problem, how can it be part of the solution? Research shows that the act of dieting increases your risk of gaining weight so in order to find peace with food, you have to reject the idea that there are any good diets out there.[7] It's the system of dieting that is the problem; diets are a set up for failure. Get rid of books and magazines that tout diets and easy or quick weight loss. Unfollow social media accounts that propel the dieting myth and diet behaviours – especially those that make you feel bad about yourself.

HONOUR YOUR HUNGER

Reminder: hunger is a normal, biological process. Your body needs to know – and be able to trust – that it will consistently have access to food. If you try to override feelings of hunger and don't eat enough calories and carbohydrates, your body reacts with cravings and binges. Then there are the times when you were hungry and you didn't eat. Why? This too is not honouring your hunger.

MAKE PEACE WITH FOOD

Allow all foods into your diet and give yourself unconditional permission to eat whatever you want. No one food has the power to make you healthy, just as no one food has the power to make you unhealthy. When you categorise foods as good or bad or you continue to tell yourself you can't have or shouldn't have a certain food, you will eventually feel deprived; this deprivation builds into uncontrollable cravings and then potentially overeating. Why? When you finally give in to that food, you're likely to overeat – since you don't know when you'll be able to have it again. This overeating triggers guilt, which starts the cycle all over again: deprivation or restriction – cravings and overeating – feelings of guilt. I'm tired just typing this.

CASE STUDY: JULIA

Many women want peace with food and an end to yo-yo dieting or disordered eating. But the truth is, many women are trying to stop overeating without changing anything else. It doesn't work. This couldn't be more true for Julia. A real workaholic, she had her eye on the success prize her whole life. On reaching her mid-thirties, after a decade of eating on the go, depriving herself, bingeing and slowly gaining weight, she came to me for support. After the first session it became apparent that food was not the issue in Julia's life. She was lonely and exhausted and food was her comfort. I told her this and she was quick to reject my intuitive reading of her, but I had sown the seed and arranged to see her the following week. Within this time it dawned on Julia that she did indeed want to settle down and was completely overwhelmed by the process of meeting someone. A complete worker bee, she couldn't see how it was possible, where she could find the time or how she had got to this point where work was her one and only passion. Over time we worked together to guide Julia to accept the path she had taken, but be open to a new one she could create. We looked at ways she could feel nourished – away from food. She had to make peace with her life before she could make peace with food. She slowly learnt to find passions elsewhere, be open to dating, and in time she even went on a dating app. Her life became more vibrant as she stepped into her authentic self, not the Julia who saw only success in her career. She learnt to find success in other ways and in doing so she felt more satisfied. It wasn't long before she met someone and, as far as I know, they are still together today.

CHALLENGE THE FOOD POLICE

The food police are the thoughts in your head that declare you as good or bad depending on what you eat. The food police push unreasonable rules that were created by dieting and cause you to feel guilty. These rules are housed deep in your brain and pop up, often on a daily basis, to govern your food decisions. If you want to view eating foods – all foods – as normal, then you have to challenge the food police.

FEEL YOUR FULLNESS

How many of you grew up with the idea that you must eat everything on your plate? Raise your hands. For me, it was like this, and we always had dessert, so from an early age I was imprinted with a need for sweetness after anything savoury. Cue overeating! Feeling your fullness is checking in with your body to know when you are full. It's bringing more consciousness and awareness to your mealtimes.

DISCOVER THE SATISFACTION FACTOR

It's possible to be physically full but not satisfied. If you're unsatisfied you'll probably keep looking for that one thing that is going to make you feel satisfied and content, which is one of the main reasons you're likely to overeat. When you eat what you really want, the feelings of satisfaction and pleasure you get will help you be content, more often than not with less food.

COPE WITH YOUR EMOTIONS WITHOUT USING FOOD

We will come to this in the next section so I'll keep it short and sweet here. Emotional eating is very common; you are NOT alone. We often eat for reasons other than physical hunger and food is often used to cover up unpleasant feelings and emotions. It's important to find ways to comfort yourself and resolve your emotions without using food.

RESPECT YOUR BODY

As I outlined in Week 1, we are all too quick to judge ourselves and criticise our bodies. By learning to respect your body for the way it is at this moment and not trying to change it back to that of the past or an idea of how you should look in the future, you begin to live in the now and find peace. If you are too critical of your body and don't accept yourself as you are, it's hard to reject any diet mentality. Remember, self-love is true love.

EXERCISE: FEEL THE DIFFERENCE

How many of you force exercise because you think you 'should' do it? Have you ever tried reframing your thoughts around exercise to, 'maybe I could enjoy exercise'? This principle shifts your focus to the types of movement that feel good to you. Forget about the calorie-burning effect of exercise and think about how you feel after working out. Do you feel energised? Do you sleep better? If you use exercise only as a way to lose weight or eat more food, it's not going to be something you will stick with forever. I find that with clients who explore exercise, it becomes a part of them and something that keeps them in alignment with their bodies.

CASE STUDY: THE OVEREXERCISERS

This is a classic case I see time and time again. Many clients will come through my clinic doors, full of stress and anxiety and a dependence on intense exercising to keep them 'well'. When I look at their symptoms, food diaries and read into their energy levels, they are exhausted and completely running on empty. The high-intensity workouts are only fuelling their weight to stay put, or increase, as their adrenals are fighting and fatigued. Research is still ongoing on adrenal fatigue and how and why it might cause weight gain, but since the role of cortisol during stress is to provide your body with energy, you can see how it might cause an increase in appetite. I often find that many of my patients hide behind their intense workouts, whether that's through an addiction to exercise or through an inability to show weakness or a desire to blend in and look 'healthy'. Whatever the case, slowing down the pace and opting for something calmer can reap benefits, especially when trying to get to know your body. You'll feel every twinge, every emotion and be able to feel a mind–body connection. You'll be able to listen to your intuition.

HONOUR YOUR HEALTH WITH GENTLE NUTRITION

I generally describe this principle to clients like this: Think back to when you were young and you would most likely eat intuitively, eating when you were hungry and stopping when you were full. You would be heading for the garden as soon as you could to play outside and wouldn't be fussed about coming back in again until you were hungry. This isn't all of us, but many of us. Now think about what you know as an adult about nutrition. It's no surprise that you need to eat around five portions of fruits and vegetables a day, right? Fuse the intuitive inner child with adult you and you have gentle nutrition. Being healthy doesn't mean eating perfectly but it does mean considering what you eat – not too much of one thing and not too little of the other. This principle guides you to consider how certain foods make you feel, in addition to how tasty and satisfying they are to you. One meal or one snack, one day of overeating will not cause you to gain weight or have a health problem. It's not all or nothing but instead the consistency of what you eat over time.

MINDFUL EATING VERSUS INTUITIVE EATING

Before I started working in intuitive eating, I used the terms mindful eating and intuitive eating interchangeably and this isn't completely incorrect but it's well worth me noting the differences. The Center for Mindful Eating defines mindful eating as 'allowing yourself to become aware of the positive and nurturing opportunities that are available through food selection and preparation by respecting your own inner wisdom' and 'using all your senses in choosing to eat food that is both satisfying to you and nourishing to your body and becoming aware of physical hunger and satiety cues to guide your decisions to begin and end eating'. So, you can see that my take on intuitive eating does indeed include or encompass the principles of mindful eating; however, it also takes it one step further. It addresses the importance of rejecting Neggy Nancy, diet mentalities and body blocks, and respecting your body and learning self-love. Mindful eating is being aware of what you eat but intuitive eating is being aware of why and how you eat too.

WHAT INTUITIVE EATING IS NOT

You may be thinking, 'If I start to give myself permission to eat all the foods I want, I'm going to overeat.' But intuitive eating is much more than an internal food monologue. When you are so used to ignoring cues of hunger or fighting yourself to try to be in control, the alternative – i.e. allowing yourself to eat with permission – can feel like chaos. There is a nagging fear of eating all the pizza, all the biscuits or drinking all the wine – but the secret here is to learn to trust yourself to eat what you truly want. It is time to start trusting in yourself. The reality is that this choice – the choice of permission – is not chaos, it is freedom. Intuitive eating is an approach that requires time, effort and dedication. It's time to get to know your body, its signals and its hunger. It's certainly not easy, which is why I have written this book and work one-to-one with women from all around the world. But when you trust in your body, you can trust that learning to truly utilise intuitive eating as a way of life will, in time, allow a more balanced routine. You'll become body wise and body-loving.

DEALING WITH FEELINGS: EMOTIONAL EATING

I want to start this section by stating that I see you and I hear you. I don't know anyone, from clients to friends to parents, who haven't, at some point in their life, eaten emotionally. We all use food as a tool to comfort ourselves one way or another. Major life events, stress, fatigue, sadness or boredom are all triggers to eat emotionally. Beat, the eating disorders charity, carried out a national survey into emotional overeating: 85 per cent of respondents said they have a negative body image; 79 per cent felt pressure from society to lose weight.[8] Emotional eating is real. So how do you determine whether you eat emotionally or not?

ARE YOU AN EMOTIONAL EATER?

- Do you eat more when you're feeling stressed?
- Do you eat when you're not hungry or when you're full?
- Do you eat to feel better (to calm and soothe yourself when you're sad, mad, bored, anxious, etc.)?
- Do you reward yourself with food?
- Do you regularly eat until you've stuffed yourself?
- Does food make you feel safe? Do you feel like food is a friend?
- Do you feel powerless or out of control around food?

Emotional eating gets a bad rep but it's actually a great way for the body and mind to prompt you that something is wrong. It's a clue that something needs addressing and a coping mechanism just like any other. Sometimes we really do need to satisfy our emotional needs and that's okay, but it's when we repeat this cycle and overuse this coping mechanism that we create harmful effects; it's the opposite of eating intuitively. When we're eating emotionally over and over again without being mindful, we're choosing to be powerless. We're choosing to be powerless by going into what I call food ecstasy; everything is great, you zone out and, by switching off the mind, you forget what was bothering you in the first place. You become focused solely on the pleasure of the food you're eating. Until . . . the second you're done indulging, you come back into reality, the good feelings disappear, and you're left feeling guilty and regretful. Ring any bells? Emotional eating only suppresses our feelings; it doesn't change them. It's like a cold caller who keeps on until you ask to be taken off the calling list. You need to take action to improve the situation. You want to be powerful. The key is getting specific about what's bothering you.

FACING YOUR STUFF – NOT STUFFING YOUR FACE

So what happens if you find you are eating emotionally? I'm a big fan of asking questions, as by doing so, you can identify and then, in turn, change your perspective.

If you realise you're about to eat emotionally, ask yourself:

1. What's really bothering me? Or what am I really hungry for?
2. What can I do about it?
3. Why don't I do anything about it? (This is the kicker: are you keeping yourself stuck?)

Think about how you talk to yourself. Instead of saying, 'I'm so stressed', try asking yourself why: 'I'm so stressed because I need to speak to my boss about a pay rise but I'm scared' or, 'I'm so stressed because of the argument I had with my partner this morning.' The more we can pinpoint what's bothering us and then take action to resolve the issue, the fewer cravings and urges we'll have. The only way to get over emotional eating is by getting to the root cause of the emotions. It's facing our stuff, NOT stuffing our face. Without a foundation of what needs to change, be addressed or be dealt with, our efforts to withdraw from emotional eating are a waste of time. This is why diets don't work over the long term; they don't change habits and behaviours. They don't focus on the mindset. Here's how to get to grips with your stuff.

NO MORE FRIDGE FILL

If you have a tendency to stand in front of the fridge and pick at foods, the first step towards reducing this emotional eating is to stop yourself anytime you feel a binge coming on and analyse your feelings by asking yourself the hunger questions below to determine whether your hunger is originating in your stomach or your mind. Instead of mindlessly running off to the kitchen, take a few minutes to think about your hunger and establish whether its origin is emotional or physical.

Am I really hungry, or am I just a creature of habit?

Unnecessary eating can hinder your progress in eating intuitively as you try to fight with the signals your body is giving you. For example, do you eat at 4pm because, in your mind, that is when snack time is? Is this a habit and are you really hungry? Instead of focusing on food, give yourself a managing strategy. There are two tactics clients of mine have found most useful: one is pressing the thumb and index finger together and saying in their mind's eye, 'I'm in control.' Secondly, if you find yourself wandering to the fridge yet again, speak out loud to yourself: 'I am walking to the fridge again to eat more food.' It sounds funny and it is. In doing so you give yourself a sharp realisation that you aren't in fact hungry at all.

Am I really hungry, or am I devouring one imprint over and over?

You can identify this type of hunger by paying special attention to your cravings and the story behind them. Have you always told yourself you need chocolate during your period or on Fridays or after a bad day at work? This is an emotion talking via your imprint. It's the same story going over and over again. Can you think of a way to shake up this story? Simply becoming aware and telling yourself that you no longer live with this imprint is enough.

Am I really hungry, or am I sleep deprived and stressed?

Studies tie your hunger to the hormone ghrelin, which rises with a lack of sleep and an increase in stress.[9] Elevated levels of ghrelin make you feel ravenous and the foods you crave are typically sugar, fats and those rich in calories. When we sleep, we are in a state of fasting because our bodies stop sending hunger signals, which would only disturb our sleep. Sleep allows your system to return ghrelin levels back to normal and, in turn, your hunger levels to normalise. Try to go to bed earlier at night, and keep track of any changes in your hunger levels and how you eat emotionally.

Am I really hungry, or am I bored?

A friend used to say to me, 'If you're bored of London, you're bored of life.' Well, I don't live in London now but I agree with the quote. Look at the world around you. How is there time to be bored? If boredom is your thing, you'll enjoy Week 5, where we look at how to feel satisfied. I'll leave this here.

KNOW YOUR TRIGGERS

To move away from eating emotionally, discover your triggers and make a plan. When you know your triggers, you can be prepared. If you know you eat when you're lonely, plan to call a friend or make a date to do something. Emotional eating can be your body's reaction to feeling deprived, so perhaps try carrying food with you or create new ways to nourish yourself. Stock your fridge with delicious foods, pack your calendar with exciting things to do, and be disciplined about setting aside time for yourself to relax.

The T-R-U-T-H technique was devised by Tina Gilbertson in her book *Constructive Wallowing: How to Beat Bad Feelings by Letting Yourself Have Them*. It's a way to let bad feelings move through you, so that you can get back to a state of calm after the upset. It also allows you to tackle your emotions head-on before you indulge in something which might in turn make you feel guilty, such as emotional eating.

T – Tell yourself the situation

R – Realise what you're feeling

U – Uncover self-criticism

T – Try to understand yourself

H – Have the feeling

Use your journal here if you need to.

USE A ROUTINE

Contrary to what I've said before, some of you may find a routine works for you. If you're a constant grazer, is it that perhaps you need to explore eating three solid meals a day in order to feel satisfied? If you're over-eating because you aren't consuming enough during the day, then getting yourself into a routine can help. Or perhaps, if boredom is the trigger, you need a night-time routine that keeps you busy and away from the fridge. Rituals and routines can be a huge support in overcoming emotional eating or setting you up for the day. A mindful morning can result in a mindful day, and research has revealed that mindfulness shows promise for improving eating patterns and a cortisol response.[10]

STRESS SOS

What are your current coping mechanisms? We all feel tough emotions from time to time, like frustration, anxiety, loneliness or boredom, but it's important to realise that food can't actually fix any of these feelings or solve problems in your life. Try finding new appropriate outlets for uncomfortable emotions and stress. Try exercising in a fun way, meditation, writing a journal, massage therapy, acupuncture, or spending time with people you love. You know the tools; it's up to you to use them. This comes back to knowing that you are the centre of your universe and that, without keeping yourself topped up, you are only perpetuating the problem.

DON'T ABANDON YOURSELF

Emotional eating provides a release from discomfort, delivering a momentary sense of pleasure and satisfaction when you're feeling something you don't want to feel. Overeating has a numbing, softening effect on our unwanted sentiments, and takes our attention away from them. The key to ending this pattern is to not abandon yourself when your emotions go awry, but instead to invite them in and allow yourself to feel. If you're feeling emotional, allow yourself to feel those feelings. In the privacy of your own heart, you can always take your side. Tell yourself that it's okay to feel sad, mad, scared or tired. Welcome your negative emotions with kindness and curiosity, and ask them what they want from you. This includes those intense feelings of guilt or anger that tend to follow an emotional-eating episode. When you approach your feelings with kindness, your body will begin to understand and trust that it no longer has to overeat to protect you from your feelings. Plus, through listening to your emotions, you'll discover what it is you truly want, and in turn you can create new strategies for deeper satisfaction.

It's time to wake up to your beauty and feed your body with the love and compassion it deserves. You are unique, beautiful and rich in resources. You have the key to satisfaction and a life without denial. When you wake up to you, you needn't deny yourself food to try to change yourself. You wouldn't need to eat emotionally as a release, because there'd be no tension to release. When you own who you are, you allow any shift in diet to be from self-love and care for your body, and not because the culture around you is dictating how you should feel and be in your skin. Own who you are and wake up to your own beauty.

DEALING WITH FRIENDS:
SOCIAL OCCASIONS

When trying to listen to your body and eat intuitively, peer pressure can be a real struggle. There may always be someone judging your choices, or trying to pressure you to eat something because it makes them feel better about themselves. I've been there on numerous occasions and so I felt it imperative to include a guide on this in the book.

Over the years, I've found that, for many women, there is a certain amount of shame around how they eat and how they feel about their bodies. If they have an addictive relationship with food, it can be hidden given that the one characteristic that makes food addiction so unique is that humans cannot live without food! If there's body-shaming, it's so easily disguised as acceptable now, as most women talk so negatively about their bodies. It's become the norm. The world is becoming increasingly designed to make us feel flawed. How do advertisers make you want to lose weight? By trying to highlight your imperfections. How do you get someone to buy into anti-ageing products? You make them worry about growing older. Then there's the constant comparison and judgement around diet. Some people will judge or do their best to have you fall off the wagon because they are insecure. People who are insecure are generally afraid of change, even if that change doesn't affect them directly. For an insecure person, someone doing better for themselves will make them feel worse about their own situation, so they'll do whatever they can to discourage you and kill your spirit. This is time for YOU. Trust that you are not alone and that there is nothing to be ashamed about. Your body is unique and if we weren't fed so much nonsense around what we should be striving for in terms of looks and health, we'd be celebrating our bodies, not bashing them. Now is the time to find your own intuitive path, your way.

I've found that when you first embark on learning the intuitive eating process, it's better to keep it to yourself. People around you may want to have their say, judge you or be keen to know more, which, at this point, might be difficult for you to share. Coming to terms with your own diet mentalities and body blocks will need time, self-care and trust in yourself; this is new territory, after all. There's always a certain expectation of how you'll be at the dinner table or a party. You will not always be on the same page as those who surround you, so make a choice based on where you are. Trying to please other people will only throw off your natural hunger and fullness cues and leave you more confused.

OWN YOUR JOURNEY

No one is with you 24 hours a day and no one else has to live in your body. If your friend or partner is begging you to share dessert but you are already full and know you really don't want it, say no. If you want dessert but your friend does not, eat it. If you want steak while your company eats a salad, enjoy it. If you are not hungry at a party, you don't need to eat the canapés. If someone brings on the guilt for not eating everything on your plate when there are starving children in Africa, why not make a donation that will actually get food where it needs to go? You know you better than anyone else and it's okay to say NO. Eating out of food peer pressure that ends up leaving you feeling full and uncomfortable is not okay. Finishing your plate does not feed the poor. Pick your battles. Most importantly, denying yourself food because someone else is not hungry will leave you starving and only at risk of bingeing later. Own your journey.

If you need to find new inspiration on your journey, learn from the habits of other people who have been successful in what you're trying to accomplish, and focus on applying those habits to your own life. Follow social media accounts that inject life and positivity into you, rather than gearing up your comparison. Join a class, read a new style of book, whatever it takes to find new inspiration.

STRENGTHEN TRUST IN YOURSELF

Trust yourself and have confidence in your body. When you know deeply what feels good to you, it's harder for things to sway you. Try writing down in the notes section on your phone how you want to feel about your food choices and your body. Whenever you feel wobbly, or someone sends you into a panic of self-loathing or body-shaming, retrieve the note, read it aloud and bring that feeling back into your body. It always makes me laugh how people think it is appropriate to comment on your diet choices, and it happens a lot. You can't control what people say, but you can control how you react to it. I've found the greatest strength comes from trusting in yourself and trying not to engage. The power of your mind is everything. Trusting yourself makes you rock solid in your choices. Over time it becomes easier not to react on emotion. Trust that you know your body better than anyone else.

Finally . . . remember that everyone has their own story to deal with. You never know what people are going through in their own heads, but often it can be the reason why they make a judgement on you. As you shift the conversation in your own head to what is best for you and your body, you can start to remove the emotion, leading you to make choices without clouded judgement. You'll learn to honour your own body and, over time, food peer pressure stops being a screaming in your ear and more white noise in the background.

FEED YOUR SOUL: THE TOOLKIT

How are you feeling about food now? Do you feel ready to start including the Intuitive Eating principles into your life? Begin small and implement something new each week. This is a journey and these tools encourage you to get to know what foods feed your soul. It's time to get to know food. Once you overcome the idea of good and bad food, the world is your oyster. It's time to celebrate food and find pleasure in everything it has to offer.

GET CREATIVE

If you want to be inspired by food, you need to get into an inspired place, feng shui-style. The kitchen is the space in the house that nourishes you and sustains life. In feng shui, it represents wealth and prosperity. Clean out the cupboards, label your dry goods and tidy your drawers; it's time to get creative in the kitchen. I love having pots of fresh herbs on the windowsill, colourful fruits in the fruit bowl and a heavily labelled and easily navigated kitchen. Inspire yourself. De-cluttering your kitchen can be a great way to start. Ready to cook something new? Cooking is a sense memory tool and gives you the ability to slow down, appreciate your food and your body. Take time with cooking this week and journal if anything comes up. Have you discovered anything about yourself? If you don't like cooking alone then invite friends over and cook for them or spend a Saturday in the kitchen with your flatmate, partner or a parent. Give yourself permission to cook something that you really love. It could be a meal you remember from your childhood, or something you never allow yourself because of a diet mentality. Make a social gathering of it, let go and enjoy.

GIVE YOURSELF PERMISSION

The goal of weight loss should be put permanently on the back burner. This is a time to give yourself permission. Permission to eat. Permission to try something new. Permission to live. The motivation of wanting to lose weight to look better, especially for a specific event, can be temporary and fleeting – but, as we've established, it has a damaging effect both psychically and emotionally. Recognise the importance of giving to your body. How does this nourish your mind? Give your body what it needs, whether that's to nourish feelings, assuage fatigue or mitigate what feels like a lifetime of deprivation.

RELEASE FORBIDDEN FOODS

It's absolutely true that some foods are more nutrient-dense than others, but vowing to eliminate certain foods or food groups from your diet forever can just increase feelings of preoccupation with forbidden foods. Eating intuitively encourages you to make peace with food. Stop with the good, the bad, the superfoods and the junk foods and make all foods equal. Stop expecting perfection or the assumption you'll never have your favourite comfort foods again. You will. Remember that all foods fit and what you need each day will be different from the next. If you often use food as a reward, write a list of other things that bring you joy and make you feel rewarded. Use these instead of food for one week and see how you feel. Does taking ten minutes each morning to read pages of your book feel better than eating a piece of chocolate? Keep in mind that making healthy choices is a way of practising self-care. Food is not a reward, just like exercise is not a punishment. They are both ways of caring for your body and helping you feel your best. You deserve both.

Now that you've tackled the intuitive eating side of intuitive living, you are ready to be taken onto the path of satisfaction. Welcome to Week 5: finding satisfaction.

Finding Satisfaction

UNDERSTANDING SATISFACTION

Satisfaction is my favourite subject. I believe that finding satisfaction is the driving force and the key to a happy life. It's also the driving force behind living intuitively, rich with a mind–body connection. Imagine it like this: everything around you represents the spokes of a wheel but the wheel itself is the satisfaction. You get to choose the number of rods radiating from the centre of the wheel. You get to choose their colour, their density and their strength. Life is the hub where the spokes connect. In this chapter we'll explore how we find satisfaction with food but, also, how to feel more satisfied with life. This is your time. Living intuitively is living the life you want to live, not the one you think you 'should' live. You've just learnt the foundation of your journey with intuitive eating so now, when you give yourself some grace and flexibility in your food choices, when you eat the pizza base and the full-fat cheese you're craving instead of greens, you're slowly but surely learning to satisfy your soul with food. Now I'm guiding you to feel satisfied with the simple pleasures in life. Sound good?

It's funny, as I was writing this chapter I started my mornings as I do every day, by watching the news with my family while eating breakfast. I've realised recently that I actually don't like watching the news anymore. I'm all for understanding where we are politically, of course, but it seems like every day is full of dark stories and negativity, which I feel completely powerless to support. What a way to start the day. A daily sense of social burden is not how I thrive and live authentically. It got me thinking about control. Just like we control what stories we imprint on ourselves from others and what we scroll on our screens, we have complete control over what we choose to do in order to feel satisfied.

As I've explained, in the realms of disordered eating food is rarely the issue, but more of a crutch to deal with an underlying problem; usually a lack of satisfaction in an area of life. When it comes to body image, once we learn to feel satisfied with all areas of our life, we take the emphasis away from striving for this unattainable perfection or 'perfect' body. When we feel out of alignment in life, we aren't utilising our intuition. When we understand the richness and ease of satisfaction in life, we bring ourselves into the sphere of intuitive living. We learn to understand what it means to feel truly satisfied. Satisfaction can come in so many forms. I've shared with you the importance of taking time for yourself, resting, eating, reading – whatever it is that makes you feel good about life, and good about you. But let's get to the nitty-gritty of *your* satisfaction, shall we. Take your journal and answer these questions:

- What does satisfaction mean to you? How would you define it?
- What does it feel like when you know you are satisfied?
- What does it feel like in your body?
- What emotional feelings come up for you when you think about satisfaction?
- What would it take to feel satisfied?

SATISFACTION COMES FROM WITHIN

The key to understanding how to feel satisfied is to trust that it comes from within.

Let's imagine you receive praise at work for your accomplishments. It could make you feel a sense of acknowledgement today, but what if tomorrow you go unrecognised and, instead, make a mistake? Would this completely erase the praise of yesterday, or make you feel like your experience is invaluable? Let's bring food into the equation. Perhaps you have what you deem a 'good' day or week and lose some weight and someone comments on your achievement. A few weeks down the line you regain the weight, but no one comments because, of course, in our crazy society we couldn't and wouldn't ever comment that someone had actually put on weight! Internally, perhaps you are waiting for someone to say that you look better with the weight back on but, if that day never comes, you will continue to internalise the inner dialogue, the drip, drip, drip that says you haven't accomplished. The likelihood is you'll jump back on the diet bandwagon so that you can receive this praise again. The cycle continues.

The acclaim of others is wonderful, but it is no marker for success and your individual satisfaction. It's equally important that you feel good about your work and trust that you are doing your best. Though outside praise may be nice and lift you up temporarily, it is not necessary for you to strengthen your own sense of self-worth. It's this self-worth that keeps you topped up with satisfaction. Appreciating and praising your own success for how it makes you feel, rather than the praise you get from others, adds a whole new dimension to the idea of satisfaction. The admiration of other people will mean so much more when you are able to think highly of yourself. Turn your gaze inwards and allow yourself to value your own triumphs. Your best is always good enough, because it comes from you, and you are always good enough.

SATISFACTION VERSUS HAPPINESS

The words happiness and satisfaction may have a similar meaning to you, but in the world of intuitive living they are very different. Before you begin to look at how satisfaction allows an intuitive life it's important for you to know the difference between satisfaction and happiness. In a nutshell, the word happiness describes a state of pleasure – like that which we get from food, a full-bodied *vin rouge* or a fleeting moment of intense elation. Satisfaction is a state of contentment and takes a much deeper, personal investment. Often things that don't make you feel happy at the time end up giving you the greatest satisfaction. For example, my training as a nutritionist wasn't always a happy time, with deadlines, exams, no spare time and a dash of stress for good measure, but I feel truly satisfied by this work and an enormous sense of achievement.

The first major study of happiness and satisfaction began in the United States in 1938, when the subject became a hot topic for research. This groundbreaking Harvard study set out to search for the key to happiness. It was originally thought that happiness could be measured objectively and externally, in much the same way as heart rate or blood pressure, but since then it has become evident that it must be measured subjectively instead, with more personal techniques including surveys, questionnaires and interviews with the subjects. Happiness is an immediate, in-the-moment experience, whereas life satisfaction is happiness that exists when we think about our lives as a whole, looking at the big picture. Based on research carried out in Europe and presented in 'The Study of Life Satisfaction', quality of life is associated with living conditions, such as food, health, shelter and so on.[1] In contrast, life satisfaction is defined as a state of emotion, like happiness or sadness. In general, whatever level of satisfaction you are feeling, you can define and maximise your wellbeing if you choose which elements you want to engage in, in order to flourish. Researchers think that roughly 40 per cent of our happiness is under our own control;[2] the rest is determined by genetics and external factors. This means there is a huge amount that you can do to control your happiness. Other research has shown that there are three main things that make people happy: close relationships;[3] both a job and a hobby that they love;[4] and helping others.[5]

To look at life satisfaction, we must consider variables such as mental and physical health, energy, self-compassion and self-worth. In intuitive living, it is based on your own cognitive judgements of the elements that you yourself consider to be valuable. Establishing a satisfying life for yourself is not decided only by circumstances, but is also influenced by the way you think about and relate to the world around you. To live life satisfied, you must, for example, consider all of the following factors:

- Collective action: action taken together by a group of people. This is your sense of belonging in a community and how you collectively work to a common goal. This is also the actions you take as an individual and how they impact your community.
- Individual behaviour: your personal attitude, perception and personality. How you hold yourself, choose your beliefs and demonstrate them.
- Simple sensory experiences: what you feel with your physical senses. How connected you are to your senses and how you interpret them.
- Higher self: how connected you are to your spirit, the self, your intuition.
- The environment: your environment, from your home to your office and on a wider scale, locally and globally.
- Chance factors: magic or chance moments, how you interpret them and how or if you allow them to guide you in life.

TASK: SATISFACTION PLAN

With this in mind, put pen to paper and, without intention or judgement, write down what satisfaction means to you. Can you pinpoint what makes you happy versus what makes you satisfied? Bring into mind all of the above factors – are there more that stand out to you or things that perhaps you've realised you haven't tapped into for a while? Is there a direct link between an area of dissatisfaction and your relationship with your body or food? Are you giving enough to others, or perhaps you aren't giving enough to yourself? Reflect on this before we move on to the following sections and, remember, there is no right or wrong. This is simply a time for you to get to know you and re-establish your mind–body connection.

SIMPLIFY: ONE THING AT A TIME

While you may feel like a multitasking machine, I'll pose the question: could life be more satisfying if you did one thing at a time? I completely understand you may all have to-do lists coming out of your beautiful bottoms, but we don't need to do them all at once. Is simplifying your day and working through each task one by one going to help you feel satisfied with what you've achieved? I guarantee it will help. When I'm writing, I turn my phone and email notifications OFF. This leaves me free of distractions to get my writing done, keep me in the zone and on schedule.

To be happy, you have to find yourself first and know who you are and what you want to be. Then you become open to discovering the things that really matter to you and, in turn, what truly makes you feel satisfied. I welcome you to this journey. You might not get answers today or tomorrow, maybe not even next week. But now you are open and on the path to intuitive living, aka satisfaction. Sometimes satisfaction can come from the little things. I often work from home and looking up from my computer to see flowers brings me absolute joy. Having a tidy workspace without clutter keeps me sane and satisfied with the work I get done. Take time to think about what simple things bring you joy and make each day more special. It's often the little shifts that have the biggest impact. So what little things around the house or the office can have the greatest impact? Now let's look at what is stopping you.

I CAN'T GET NO, SATISFACTION

Whether satisfaction seems completely out of reach, or something that has momentarily been forgotten, it's important that you understand where it may have gone and why. In this section we'll look at what could be keeping you small and dissatisfied in life. Can you remember a time in your life when you felt fully committed to pursuing your passion? Every single cell in your body felt rich in its resources, and focused on this passion. Then, there may be other times when necessity or some kind of responsibility directed you to put your dreams on hold for a while. Maybe this while turned into months, or even years. Over this time you may have forgotten or lost what it was that you really loved to do. Maybe you know exactly what it is but you feel that with the process of 'adulting', aka growing up, there isn't space in your life for this anymore.

There are many reasons why we leave our passions behind. A hobby can lose its appeal if attempts to make it a career don't work out. Time constraints can make a hobby seem impossible, especially when work is busy and life gets in the way. Maybe you embark on parenthood, which turns everything upside down and you feel there is no time to continue doing things you once loved. You might be thinking, where is time for me?! Or perhaps it is someone else who got in your way. Someone important to you might have always told you that your passion is unsuit-able for a long-term life goal or career. Maybe this became imprinted on your subconscious; you weren't good enough, confident enough, smart enough. Maybe you started to believe them.

Perhaps you've neglected your passion because you felt there were too many other responsibilities taking centre stage. Or you felt there was an order in which things needed to happen and that time for yourself and your dreams would come once you got everything else out of the way. There is no need to neglect your responsibilities in order to pursue a passion, just as you don't have to neglect your commitments to do something that brings you satisfaction and joy. There is room for both yet I can't tell you how many times I've seen these pesky beliefs come up. The problem is, they are usually false. There are no rules to getting on and playing big. You don't need to wait until there is time to learn the language before moving to the country you desire to live in. Nine times out of ten your belief will be a story you've created to keep you in your comfort zone. When you make an effort to incorporate both your responsibilities and your desires into your life, you allow the fire within you to ignite.

YOUR FOCUS IS YOUR SUPERPOWER

I feel like I'm about to tell you something that is going to change your life forever. The more you focus on things outside of your body, the more you feel at home in it. When we forget about what we love doing – our passions and our hobbies – it is, to our mind and body, a form of self-sabotage. When we move the focus outside of our bodies, we open up a world of time, energy and possibilities. We open ourselves up to feeling satisfied. Just because things didn't work out or it felt out of reach for a short while, it doesn't mean you have to forget about your dreams. It doesn't mean that they no longer exist. They may just take a new form. Think back to hobbies that you've left behind. If you feel like you've forgotten, think about what activities you loved as a child or interests you used to have. Did you play an instrument or have something you wished you'd explored but never quite got round to it? What has filled that space since? Nothing fills the void of a passion that has been tossed aside. Let me ask you now, what's stopping you? What is preventing you from picking up that guitar or enrolling in that drawing class? Life is too short to stop doing what brings you joy and satisfaction.

WALKING ON THE WILD SIDE: RISKING FAILURE

I've found with many of my clients that they've forgotten about their dreams because that means they would never have to risk failure. For many of them growing up, failure was not an option. From childhood into adulthood they were so scared of failing that they got into the mindset of playing it safe. They would find solace in food. It's so easy to get tangled up with the idea of being the best: the best child, the best parent, the best employee, having the best body or the best diet. But isn't it boring being the best? With failure comes wisdom. When we try to be the best, we run the risk of short-circuiting any of our originality and uniqueness, because, of course, we are only striving to fit into someone else's vision of success. We don't jump outside of the box. If everyone were striving for the same outcome, what a boring world it would be; we'd lose out on creativity and diversity. I'm not saying here that we shouldn't want to improve and, of course, examining others can give us inspiration – but trying to be the best can be exhausting and who decides what's 'best' anyway?

SHOWING UP FOR YOURSELF

Once again, it's time to let go. If fear is standing in the way of your satisfaction, try to list what beliefs you have and how you hold yourself to other people's standards. When you let go of the belief that you need to compete and win and, instead, adopt a mindset whereby you own your sh*t and trust that you're doing the best job you can, you begin to show up for yourself. You strive to do your best. You create a life free of regret, knowing you've performed to the best of your ability, which allows you to feel a greater sense of satisfaction in your efforts, regardless of how others may have perceived the outcome. Showing up for yourself encourages you to get to know yourself and be open to learning from your past and current endeavours. Typically, when I introduce women to the way they hide from themselves and keep themselves small, they have incredible 'aha' moments. I ask every single client I see what vision they hold for themselves in their life and health. Then, I ask them what's stopping them feeling this way now, today. Bring to mind reasons why you don't feel satisfied; create a list. Now think of the reasons for this. Is it because you lost the desire or responsibilities took over? Now, next to each one, note down what is stopping you from feeling that way again. Here's an example:

CASE STUDY: OLIVIA

In her vision, Olivia saw herself in a beautiful dress, confident, sexy and vibrant. She feels alive in her body. She is creative and living more in her artist side versus the work she is currently doing, which she has taken on for financial reasons. When I asked Olivia what was stopping her feeling this way now, she explained that she knew she has a 'f**k it' attitude. She was a little lazy and couldn't be bothered to honour her body and desires. When we delved deeper, it turned out that Olivia viewed being attractive as hard work, therefore she felt she didn't have the energy to embark on such a journey. She also admitted to being quite the perfectionist and to feeling like she had to lower her expectations of herself to take her away from being all or nothing. Session by session we broke down these barriers, first by reframing what attractive meant and empowering her to see her own attractiveness. We then worked on the disassociation of attractiveness with hard work and, on a practical level, found time for her to look after herself. In time she began to step into that vision until, eventually, she became her future self, her ideal and authentic self.

CENTERING YOUR OWN DESIRES

This might seem like a radical act but if you want to feel satisfied, you need to start centering your own desires. Your sense of purpose has greater impact than the fears surrounding it. Being able to recognise and pursue what it is that makes you feel satisfied is a fundamental human right. Own it. If you've been feeling out of touch with your own wants for years, think about where you can regain them. If food comes into play here and you've been using it as a way to feel satisfied, know that much of this is through the course of living in a diet culture-heavy society. You've been so bombarded with the message that what you want to eat, how you want to move your body, how you want to take pleasure from things outside the norm is wrong. Maybe you've started to second-guess your intuition and stop knowing what you actually want. Now it's time to start centring your own desires and getting clear on what brings you peace, with both food and your body, and your life. Start to reconnect with the desires that have always been there, and to see that those desires are trustworthy. Turn on your inner wisdom, the one you were born with, and allow this trust to create a ripple effect throughout your life.

TASTE SENSATION

Think back to your earliest memory of food. Can you describe the textures, the flavours, the smell? If I asked you what your favourite meal was, could you remember? What about the last meal you'd want to eat before you die? Many cultures appreciate the time to sit and savour food. They take pleasure in it. They give it a dedicated hour, sometimes two. In many cultures there is nothing 'low fat' on the shelves. In our culture, it's everywhere. On-the-go meals, drive-thru food chains, pre-packed everything; it's easy for us to have lost the love for food. And, of course, without taking the time to savour food, how can it really, truly satisfy you? Isn't that what food deserves? Isn't that what you and your body deserve? This section focuses on taste sensations – why and how we've lost feeling satisfied from foods and how to get the feeling back.

EATING BEHAVIOURS

How we eat now has a lot to do with how we ate as a child. In her book *First Bite: How We Learn to Eat*, Bee Wilson explains that what the mother eats, the baby gets a taste of, through her breast milk. Eating behaviours then evolve during the first few years of life, when children learn what to eat, when and how much – through intuition, yes, but also through experiences with food and by observing the eating patterns and behaviours of others. It's these observations that are most challenging for my clients. Here are the key behaviours I see them pick up:

- Watching parents dieting
- Mothers or siblings with disordered eating/eating disorders
- Father being overly critical of the mother's intake of food, or his own
- Both parents being overly fearful of the child's weight and, in the case of some, being sent to weight-loss camps or diet support groups such as Slimming World or Weight Watchers
- Being around fussy eaters

By the time these women move into adulthood, their eating patterns have been highly shaped by what they picked up in their youth. Many end up living exactly like their mothers, constantly dieting. Or they still binge as a way to rebel against a controlling father. The cycle continues into adult life.

It's been thoroughly researched that restriction of children's access to and intake of foods can at that time and in later life promote an overconsumption of these once-restricted foods when they are readily available.[6] Children with a highly restricted diet have poor self-regulation of energy intake, which is associated with greater weight gain across childhood and into adult life.[7] There have been recent studies to show that children who help cook at home are more likely to enjoy fruits and veggies than kids who don't cook at all.[8] Seeing is believing, you might say. It's also been shown that, in adult life, overeating in the absence of food deprivation only perpetuates a cycle of overconsumption and one that resembles, both behaviourally and neurochemically, a pattern of addiction.[9]

So, what we know is that with food restriction we see bouts of over-eating, but what exactly is it about food that makes us feel satisfied, or simply momentarily satisfied, as I see in my clinic . . . ?

WHY FAT IS YOUR FRIEND

When your tongue comes into contact with food, taste receptors are acti-vated and signals are sent to your brain, which then helps to regulate your intake. It takes 20 minutes for your stomach to signal to your brain that it's full, so when we eat quickly, we lose this signal until we've over-eaten. When a low-fat version of your favourite food hits your tongue, your brain and digestive system never quite get the message that they're getting something calorific and should therefore need less in order to feel satisfied. Instead, we are left with an unsatisfied feeling. Fat equals fullness! A study published in the journal *Flavour* has seen emerging evidence that may qualify fat as the sixth flavour; the first five are sweet, sour, salty, bitter and umami.[10] The fat molecule in many foods actually holds the true flavour; so when you take it out, you remove the flavour and, thus, it definitely isn't as satisfying. Plus food companies have to add something to bring back the flavour that fat offers, which is usually sugar and salt.

We need fats for more than just flavour. Vitamins A, D, E and K are fat-soluble, which means they need to be bound to fat in order for our bodies to use them. Fat acts as a transportation mechanism for fat-soluble vitamins in the body. All of these vitamins play an important role; being deficient in any comes with health consequences. For example, vitamin D deficiency is implicated in the increase in the incidence of rickets in the UK since the mid-1990s.[11] Dietary fat also helps maintain your body temperature, insulates your organs, supports hormone production and cell growth, and gives you energy. Fat for fuel and your body; it's kind of important.

Eating can often feel like a Catch-22: to reach the ultimate satisfaction with food, feelings of guilt should be minimal or nonexistent following food intake; however, we often eat based on how we feel at that moment, and on how certain foods affect the way we feel. We eat because we are emotional, but we are then consumed with guilt from eating foods purely to deal with our feelings. To learn to be satisfied, feelings of pleasure and fulfilment outside of food have a huge impact; when your wishes or needs are met, there is less emphasis on food to make you happy.

WHY DO WE EAT?

We fill our bodies with food to prevent hunger, which is the body's natural urge to eat. An urge can stem from a want or need for food or from something more intense – a strong desire or craving. Food influences and choices can include the following factors:

- Environmental: convenience and availability of food in a certain area or environment
- Familial: familiar foods and meals consumed while living at home and eating with family
- Social: choices based on health trends or in conjunction with social groups of friends, co-workers, classmates, etc.

- Cultural: eating habits and preferences based on a particular group, time, place or society
- Individual: foods chosen based on personal taste, want and feelings

With such a wide variety of food influences, you might be asking how do you go about feeling satisfaction from food? Now, firstly, satisfaction varies from person to person. For some of you, a home-cooked meal with family and friends might bring you all the joy; however, for others, it's taking a bath with a pack of Dairy Milk after a long and stressful day. But the secret to feeling satisfied simply from food is to reach a place where guilt post-consumption is either minimal or completely nonexistent.

GOODBYE GUILT

The consumption of food can be a vicious cycle. For example, you need a snack and you choose an apple because an apple is deemed 'healthy'. The apple doesn't satisfy you so you try a vegan nut-and-date bar. You're still unsatisfied. Finally, you fill the void with a brownie, which was really what you wanted in the first place, but because you have eaten the apple and the nut bar as well, you now feel overly full. There is instant satisfaction but this is followed by guilt and shame. Does this resonate with you? Can you imagine a world in which you allow yourself the brownie in the first place without guilt and shame? It is possible. Staying in tune with your hunger and satiety is key. The body has a response – the 'I'm full' sensation – which you must honour. Plus, learning the benefits of all foods you are eating – from emotional support through to fats for fat-soluble vitamin transportation – can help to build a positive relationship with the food you consume, based upon health and wellness versus shame and guilt.

CASE STUDY: CARRIE

I love cooking for people and, for a few years, I had a catering company alongside my nutrition practice. One year I was cooking on a retreat and one of the teachers who came along announced she wouldn't be eating my food and instead would be making her own; a juice cleanse, she said. Every day I saw her make her green smoothies and juices, while I and the other teachers and guests dived into delicious meals – chia puddings, Birchers, salads, stews, barbecued fish and cacao puddings. I couldn't help but notice that Carrie would head to the kitchen while we were eating outside, enjoying wine and conversation. She would be making herself a small plate, then going back for more and more until she had eaten a full-size meal, often more than the other guests. Now, you see, what Carrie wanted was to deprive herself in order to lose a few pounds on the trip or feel 'cleansed' by limiting foods. But with this deprivation she wasn't at all satisfied and so ended up eating exactly what we were all eating, often more, but instead of celebrating with food and friends, she ate alone and in secret. How things could have been different for her had she allowed herself to be more mindful and enjoy the surroundings, the people, the food. The moral of this story is that food should be celebrated and, when we eat for pleasure, we can feel much more satisfied.

HOW TO FEEL SATISFIED FROM FOOD

DYNAMIC CONTRAST

Food pleasure is a combination of sensory factors (sensation) and caloric stimulation by the macronutrients (protein, carbohydrates and fat). Aroma is also important in food, as is texture. What food combinations make you go ooooh? What flavours, cuisines, aromas and textures turn you on? As a general rule of thumb, satisfying meals contain fat, protein and carbohydrates. While high-volume or low-calorie foods may signal fullness by filling up your stomach, fat, protein and carbohydrates all signal fullness in other ways, i.e. by bringing blood sugar levels back to normal or by releasing hunger-suppressing hormones. Dynamic contrast and good old macros have a big impact on our senses and, in turn, the pleasure we take from food.

PLEASURE-SEEKER

We've become so focused on the amounts, weights, pure alchemy of foods – with the aim of losing weight or seeking health – that we have forgotten a very important role of eating: to find pleasure. Do you often eat alone? Do you eat ready-made meals while sat on the sofa? Do you deprive yourself when out with friends, opting for foods you think you should order? What you put into your body has a profound, holistic effect on your emotions, so allow yourself to feel the pleasure derived from food. We're innate pleasure-seekers, and studies have shown that certain foods, such as fat, are potent natural reward-drivers.[12] When we take out the fat, the sugar, the salt, we are left with something less satisfying, and so we eat more of it, to try to feel the satisfaction. This dates back to the days of feast and famine. Our brains are programmed to desire food that gives us fuel – for survival. Nowadays, food is abundant, so instead of savouring what we eat in order to gain satisfaction, the pleasurable foods tend to be the quick-fix, on-the-go foods that we don't give enough time to. They might be full of sugar, salt or fat but we eat them so quickly, we don't even recognise the satiety. Which leads me on to . . .

SSS: SLOWLY, SENSUALLY AND SAVOUR EVERY BITE

If we don't satisfy ourselves with food, we end up longing for more – cue overeating which, let's face it, only fuels the guilt trip. To get out of the cycle, remember to eat slowly, use your senses and savour every bite. This is an easy win for my clients; it's simple to remember and encourages them back to their senses. When you eat slowly, you give your stomach time to signal to the brain you are full. When you use your senses you are mindful, aware and not distracted. When you savour every bite, you feel your satisfaction.

DON'T DISTRACT YOURSELF

Distraction is something that comes up a lot in my practice. Distracted eating is when you are aware of what you are eating, but you're distracted while you do it. Whether it is watching TV, being on the phone or working – you are distracted. Hands up who eats while being distracted? A recent study reveals the impact of eating while distracted.[13] The scientists divided people into two groups. The distracted group ate lunch while playing a computer game of solitaire and the non-distracted group ate the same lunch but without the distraction. The study proved that being distracted had a huge impact on the eating experience. The distracted people:

- Ate faster
- Couldn't remember what they ate
- Ate more snacks after the meal
- Reported feeling less full

We are living in a high-urgency, multitasking world. Even when we personally are not pressed for time, people around us are. When you eat with distractions such as texting, emailing, walking or talking, you are missing out on the eating experience. It's a bit like listening to a friend talk about her problems while emailing your boss or checking messages at the same time. Is that respectful? No. How about you take the time to listen to her, giving her your full attention, and then come back to the emails and give them your full attention later? If this feels sticky to you, ask yourself:

- Why am I resisting this?
- What would it take to be wholly present with my meals?
- What do I fear about eating in this way?

Slow the pace. Give your all to your meals. You might just feel satisfied.

FEEL YOUR FULLNESS

The importance of satisfaction is even greater than that of fullness. To explain the difference to my clients, I say that fullness is the physical sensation of satiety, while satisfaction is the mental sensation of satiety. You can be full without being satisfied. For a meal to be satisfying, it should also taste good. For example, I was at an event recently where the canapés were those 'healthy' ones; and they were pretty bad. I was hungry so I ate them. The canapés were a perfect balance of fat, protein and carbs and I ate enough to feel full, but I wasn't satisfied. So the first thing I did after the event was grab some sushi on the way home, because I still was craving satisfaction and my intuition was saying rice and fish! This is one of the reasons why diets that appear balanced still don't work – because even if you're getting enough calories and from all the food groups, if you're not satisfied, you'll still be driven to eat. I could eat a ton of raw fruit and veggies to the point where my stomach was stretched out and physically full . . . but I wouldn't feel satisfied. Who wants raw veg without a tahini and orange dressing? Not me. Without satisfaction, you'll only go on to seek it, most likely by bingeing, overeating, obsessively thinking about food or just grazing mindlessly. Satisfaction turns off the drive to eat, not fullness.

Intuitive eating is not a test; you can't pass or fail. The beauty of intuitive eating is that you have permission to get it wrong. There's so much room to experiment, get curious, and figure out what's satisfying for the unique individual that is you.

BODY SATISFACTION

Body positivity as a movement can be dated back to the Victorian era, with groups of women campaigning against society's expectation that they wear corsets. Then in the 1960s the National Association to Advance Fat Acceptance was established in the United States and campaigning turned into true activism. This is when body positivity and fat acceptance became a discussion topic, and more people started to cotton on to the idea that weight does not equal health and size discrimination is intrinsically wrong. We still have a long way to go, and I genuinely think it's wrong to imagine that we will be satisfied with our bodies every single day of the year. There may always be a window of time when you feel a bit meh and that's okay. I think it's important to admit that sometimes I myself have to dig into my own personal toolbox and find something to anchor me. In this section we are exploring body satisfaction: how to find it, embrace it and love it.

After I had my daughter, I developed acne around my chin and on my back. I felt like I was 14 again; I hated it back then, and I hated it second time round. My hair was falling out in clumps and it was really challenging to find clothes to wear that were suitable for the heat of the summer and breastfeeding – all with a spotty back. I also felt different in my body and it took time for me to feel at home in it again. I know I'm not alone in this as I've spoken with many women who have had children, operations or major illnesses who have said the same thing. No one really talks about these things post-birth. It's all about getting back 'in shape', which of course I wholeheartedly disagree with; our bodies shouldn't be expected to bounce back like an elastic band but, post-pregnancy or not, these things do affect us. What I'm getting at here is that there may be moments when you wobble, quite literally and emotionally, with your body. There are many ways to rediscover body positivity and satisfaction when it feels like it has gone astray and I've included a few of my favourites here.

INVITING IN TRUST AND LOVE

In my case, postpartum I came to the mentality that in order to ride the wave of change, I had to trust my body was doing what it needed to do. Trust the journey. I trusted that my hormones would balance. I trusted that my skin would settle. I knew that new clothes could be bought. I told my body that I still trusted it and that I respected where it was right now. Trust in the journey and trust in your body. Nothing is kinder to your body than loving it. I learnt this one from Marianne Williamson, spiritual teacher and all-round women's advocate. I adore her! It's not romantic love but instead a state of consciousness or being. At any given moment, you can invite love in. When the negative voice in your head turns to fear and tells you your body isn't worthy, strong enough, good enough, kill it with kindness and love. Say to yourself, 'I shift this negativity and turn fear into love' or, 'I bring only love and kindness to my body.' Say it over and over, breathing deeply into it as you do. There was not a single situation in which my acting more loving, compassionate and understanding would have made the situation worse. Love really always is the answer. Choose love.

HEALTH CHECK

This works as a reality check when you are on a downward spiral of body-shaming. In my practice I hear a lot of women who aspire to being 'healthy'. I ask, 'What does healthy mean to you?' Nearly always it means being lighter, slimmer, more toned. These clients will sit there praising themselves for going to the gym and eating well, yet their target and vision in life is to be healthy. But they are already healthy. They eat well, they move, they are learning daily to love themselves. It's not that they aren't healthy; it's just that their perception of what healthy means is off kilter. So whenever you are feeling this way, give yourself a reality check.

Just because you ate a piece of cake, it does not make you unhealthy. Just because you've gained weight, it does not make you unhealthy.

THE SUPERFOOD SYNDROME

A friend of mine used to work in Planet Organic, the biggest one in London. He used to get people coming in to see what was new, what the next magic superfood was that would make them 'healthy'. This is what I call the 'Superfood Syndrome' – the disorder of being obsessed with 'superfoods'! Few lies can be told in one word, but superfood manages it! Superfoods are marketed as miracle foods that will help you live longer or cure disease. But there is no one magic pill. There is no one magic superfood that is going to help you live to be a hundred. Everyone eats food, which makes it a hot topic all of the time; we all have an opinion. Of course, we are all experts on ourselves, but when it comes to superfoods much of the science doesn't support the hype. So when you are next feeling the quest for health, check in with yourself. Too much of anything isn't good for you and it doesn't have to be all or nothing. Bad science can be big money so keep your head firmly on those shoulders and don't believe the hype. Do your research. If your granny can't pronounce it, question it!

LEARN DAILY PRACTICES FOR CENTERING AND GRACE

What makes you feel centred and graceful? For me, I hate spending time getting ready. I see it as a wasted opportunity to live, so I keep a simple hair style that needs very little upkeep. I wear red lipstick most days because it's easy, and I wear a simple colour scheme of clothes from navy, grey and black, leaving me with more time to do the things that matter to me and reach my goals and desires. I eat well and I give myself time to prepare all of my meals because, for me, cooking is part of what makes me feel satisfied. I walk in nature every day. I treat myself like a goddess every day. I don't deprive myself. I laugh. I know it isn't easy and sometimes it takes effort – but learning your daily practices can be extremely rewarding. Regena Thomashauer, author of *Pussy* calls this 'pussification'. She talks a a lot about getting back in touch with your sexuality and it made so much sense to me. Her pleasure and satisfaction comes from dressing up and dancing. She dances her emotions in and out of her body. She goes to a dance class once a week. She masturbates regularly and has a lover who she sees frequently. The woman is incredible!

SAY THE WORD: SATISFACTION

Repeating and contemplating the word satisfaction can actually create that emotion. Say it over and over, varying the speed, tone and tempo. Notice how your body feels when you say it. Did your chest expand? Did your face relax? Did you smile? Remind yourself of what satisfaction means to you. Be as specific as possible, imagining the feeling of it, the images it conjures up, perhaps even the people and situations that trigger it. Paint the word on a rock and keep it on your desk. Stick a satisfaction memo on your fridge. Surround yourself with the word, and the more satisfaction will rise up to join you, if you simply invite it to do so.

HONOUR YOURSELF CONSCIOUSLY AND FREQUENTLY

Body satisfaction doesn't come from others; it comes from within. Interrupt negative thoughts about yourself and replace them with statements that focus on honouring yourself, such as:

- I'm fine the way I am.
- I'm whole and complete.

- I did my best.
- I can do this.
- I love myself.
- What I'm seeking is within me.

Focus on the good and what you do well. Write down self-appreciation notes so that you can read and say them frequently. The more you reinforce these concepts, the more they'll become reality.

THE WHEEL OF SATISFACTION

In the process of creating my first online six-week programme – Intuitive Eating and Living – I took a long, hard look at what made me feel satisfied, what I valued in life and how I could share this idea of satisfaction with a wider audience. The idea of happiness for me was always transient; I knew I could be unhappy for a whole day but still feel satisfied in life. As I approached 26, my life was the opposite; I had moments of happiness in among moments of unhappiness but I felt truly unsatisfied. It was at this point that I discovered I needed to outline each individual area of my life – what was important to me – and honour each part of that. This was how I came up with the idea of the Rooted Wheel of Satisfaction, which we are looking at in this section. Now that you've learnt the rules for food and body satisfaction, where can we take satisfaction further? Where do you need and want to feel satisfied in the various pieces of the life pie?

Life is full of opportunity and experience but our attention can be pulled in many different directions, not only by events in our own lives, but by advertising, the media and the hustle and bustle of our surroundings and the busy world we inhabit. When you direct the time to focus your thoughts on the goals that resonate the most strongly with you, you allow time to listen to your inner guidance. Sometimes, one area of our life needs to take centre stage – the spotlight of our attention – but this doesn't mean that we have to stay focused on only this one thing forever.

As modern life makes vast amounts of information and opportunities available to you, you might find yourself torn between a variety of interests, projects or goals. You may feel enticed to try them all, or go full throttle into one area of your life. In doing so, you may zap energy from other areas. For example, if it's all work and no play, it doesn't leave room for love, adventure or health. It leaves you unable to fully experience all of these areas of your life. When you can choose one thing at a time on which to focus all of your attention, and be conscious of other areas that need attention too, you can make the most of what life has to offer, and engage yourself fully in every moment. You can be safe in the knowledge that there is satisfaction to be had in every moment.

Here is the Wheel of Satisfaction. Look at each section: where do you feel satisfied? Have you been focused too much on one section? Are you seriously lacking in another area?

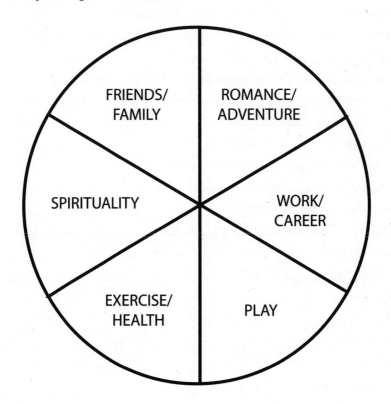

TASK: JOURNALLING

Set aside around an hour for this task. Grab your journal and list each section of the wheel down the side of the page. Now, think about what this section means to you. What is missing or not quite satisfying in this area? Then write down the following:

- What is your daily commitment to get there? (a small step, an affirmation, a thought pattern that needs to be reframed)
- What can be achieved in a month from now to reach this goal?
- What can be achieved in six months from now to reach this goal?
- What is your WOW goal in this area?

Year to year, there will be areas that feel good as they are and areas that you feel need growth. You might not have a WOW goal for everything but staying focused in each area allows you to move with the rhythmic flow of life, and check in with all aspects of your being as a balanced whole. Remember, you are multifaceted and, from moment to moment, you have different needs. Your work in the world is necessary to feel your purpose, just like how your relationships are important for your emotional needs.

Use this exercise as a way of checking in with yourself. I use mine twice a year; my own personal six-month MOT.

SATISFACTION: THE TOOLKIT

You've had the eureka moment. You know what it is to get satisfaction from food and from other areas of your life. This, dear readers, is the key to intuitive living. You've made it so far and we are so nearly there in the journey together. One question I always get asked is: what happens when I feel satisfied and then I hit a wall and fear steps on my toes? Here is my go-to toolkit for the satisfaction factor when you feel like you're having a wobble:

CREATE RITUAL

Sometimes igniting satisfaction can come in the form of a ritual. Having a daily ritual or ceremony in our lives is very important to keep us connected to what really matters to us; similar to checking in on a higher-self level. When we perform or participate in rituals and ceremonies, we enter into a state of mind that is different from our typical consciousness. Many daily rituals revolve around nourishing and cleansing, which links beautifully to food and satisfaction. Maybe it's taking a pause before each meal and closing your eyes to say a silent thank you to the universe for what it has provided. If you want to get more elaborate, try journalling on your satisfaction in a candle-lit room each week.

CHERISH FRIENDSHIPS

The Harvard study on happiness found that one of the top three things that kept us healthy and happy was our relationships.[14] The researchers found that men who reported being closer to their family, friends or community were happier and healthier than their less social counterparts. They also tended to live longer. By comparison, people who said they were lonelier reported feeling less happy. They also had worse physical and mental health. Cherish the relationships you have. Call a friend. Take a date with your loved one. Say sorry for the silly things you said. What can you do today to cultivate stronger relationships? Happiness is love and good relationships keep us happier and healthier.

CREATE YOUR WORD OF THE YEAR

Some years are about growth. Some years are about finding peace. Some years are about transformation. I love asking my clients to sum up their intentions for the year in one word. What is the one word that will guide you over the year ahead? Choosing a word for the year is so compelling because it takes the 'should' out of your own capability. This word will keep you focused and inspired. You can check in with this word when making decisions by asking, 'Does this feel (insert word of the year)?' When you open up to a word that will guide you, you're letting your intuition and your soul show you the way to a custom-made path to satisfaction. What is your word of the year?

As you awaken yourself to your satisfaction and intuition, you can become more attuned to what is right for you. The universe speaks to all of you through infinite channels, but you each have your own frequency. Only you can decide what truly makes you feel inspired, aligned, awakened, connected, fully conscious, aware and alive. Whatever your path, it is perfect and is meant especially for you.

In Week 6 you will discover how to pull together everything you've read thus far and start to create your own rules. You are the expert of your life now. The next chapter – which you might find you'll want to return to a lot – is the bring-it-all-together hotspot, with gentle reminders to keep you on the intuitive living love train along with powerful reminders for when you may have fallen off. Are you ready?

WEEK 6
Make Your Own Rules

Part One: Self-love, Body-love
Part Two: Food Rules
Rewriting Your Story: Connecting with the Future You
Transitions: Implementing Change
Manifesting Magic
Staying on the Rails: FAQs
DO YOU: The Manifesto

PART ONE: SELF-LOVE, BODY-LOVE

You've made it so far. I hope with everything you have learnt, you have realised that bad eating patterns are rarely about food. I hope you have realised that you do not have to be thin, have long hair, shave your legs, be fashionable, diet, or stay small to be worthy or to be satisfied with life. No, to live intuitively is to live with power, knowledge, confidence and trust. It shines out of you bright like a diamond. The world is ready for you. This section is a reminder on how to make your own rules around food and your body. To start with – when you're in the midst of body dys-morphic thoughts – remind yourself of this:

- Having a bigger body does not make you any less worthy of love, respect, attention or happiness.
- A number on the scales does not define your worth or your success.
- Your worth is not determined by your physical appearance.

- Getting to a certain size does not make you a better, more intelligent or successful person. You can do that at any size.
- You are so much more than your body.
- Your right weight is the weight you reach when you're living your healthiest and happiest life.
- No one is looking at you. Get out of your own head!

Most importantly, when you're too focused on getting the perfect summer body, what are you not creating? Is getting the perfect body what you were really put on this earth to do? The saying is, it's not how good you are but how good you want to be.

When I lived in my darker days of disordered eating and low self-love, I was finding my worth in the wrong things. No matter how hard I worked out, how healthily I ate, or how much I weighed, if that was what I was basing my worth on I would always come up empty. I felt defeated and alone. If only I knew then that you can change your mindset with your words. Words are everything. A growth mindset is exactly what it says, the tendency to believe that you can grow. Here's how:

1. Acknowledge and embrace imperfections. When you hide from weakness, you'll never overcome it.
2. View challenges as opportunities. What can you learn from this experience?
3. Replace 'I am failing' with 'I am learning'.
4. Stop seeking approval. Come back to your radical self-love vision. Does this experience support your self-worth?
5. Value the process, NOT the end result.
6. Reduce the reward mentality. You're neither good nor bad based on what you do, eat, say. Stop with the 'I've been good today so . . .'
7. Allow yourself time for reflection at least once a day. Keep giving back to YOU.

YOUR RADICAL SELF-LOVE VISION

Loving your body completely doesn't need to be your new goal and sole focus. We all love the idea of loving our bodies unconditionally but this stuff takes time. Be realistic by adopting a more functional view of your body – focusing on what it does for you, the skills it has and how it develops with you year on year of your life. Those with a positive body image tend to spend less time focusing on their body's outward appearance and more on appreciating and accepting the changing nature of it. This includes the emotional and mental experiences relating to embodiment. You don't need to love your body 100 per cent of the time but you can learn to accept it and have gratitude for it. Even when you're not feeling so great in it, you can really help to shape the way you think about it over time. Create a gratitude list each morning of three things that are actually having a negative impact on you, such as:

- I am grateful for the fact that I've gained weight this winter. My body knows how to keep me warm.
- I am grateful for the wrinkles on my brow, they show wisdom and strength.
- I am grateful for the stretchmarks from childhood. They remind me of how much my body changes to support me.

The goal of loving your body is different for everyone and for many it feels unattainable and unrealistic, especially if you are at the beginning stages of the idea of self-love and care. Don't give yourself a hard time. Just notice how you speak to yourself and how finding time for the little shifts can create the biggest impact. As part of the practice for self-love, you have to allow yourself to receive. It's so easy to fall back into giving and edging yourself back down to the bottom of that priority list.

What's the best compliment you've ever received? Write it down, and then spend a few minutes thinking about the words. Repeat the compliment to yourself and allow it to be received. Accept the compliment with your whole body. See yourself through a new lens. Finally, if you were fully in love with yourself, what would your life look like? How would you speak, hold yourself and move in the world? What would you do with your time and what would you cut out of your life? Take some time to daydream and create that vision. Maybe note it down in your journal. How different could your world look if you were treating yourself with nothing less than total love, self-respect and compassion?

YOUR BODY, YOUR RULES

Fill in the blanks with positive words that sing to your soul:

I love myself because . . . .
Even though I'm not perfect, my flaws make me . . . .
When I look in the mirror I see . . . .
I am comfortable in my own skin because . . . .
I take care of my body by doing . . . .
I love . . . . about my body today
I am worthy because . . . .

Say these to yourself every day. Create new ones as you develop and grow. Your body is an instrument, not an ornament. Self-love is true love.

PART TWO: FOOD RULES

My food philosophy is based on the senses, and to eat and live intuitively, senses you must use. Welcome to my rules around intuitive eating that you can reshape to work for you. Before we begin this section, ask yourself how you want food to make you feel. On my journey from diet land to diet-free living, I started breaking this down into three categories: energised, nourished and comforted. This made most sense to me, for it captured how I tend to want food to make me feel most of the time. I'll explain:

Energised: Summer loving, energised is all about fresh, sharp and zingy flavours – what you'd expect in warmer climates and in the small bursts of sunshine that we normally get in the UK summer. Energised foods are light, colourful and crisp. Think fruits, raw vegetables, crunchy leaves and fresh produce; salads, smoothies, chilled soups, sushi, poke bowls, you get my drift. What foods energise you?

Nourished: Nourishing is soul food; warm, stodgy and full of goodness. Think Indian dhals and curries, porridge, chunky soups, stews, root vegetables, anything and everything with herbs and spices from turmeric to cinnamon. Nourished is how I want to feel each winter. What foods sound nourishing to you?

Comforted: A cuddle in a mug, comforted is exactly what it says on the tin. For me comforting foods are rich, warm and often sweet – hot chocolate, rice pudding, warm creamy soups, anything with coconut milk or cream, chocolate chip biscuits, pancakes and big bowls of pasta. What is comforting food to you?

You might have other words that sum up how you like to feel from food so explore what this could mean for you. It works for many of my clients as it takes away the guessing game and gives them a clear and focused way to choose food. Food and food choices can be totally overwhelming so instead of thinking about the food itself and getting in a wobble, they can imagine how they want to feel and, from there, chose appropriately.

My thought process behind any food choice is: how will it affect my senses? When you eat, do you absorb just the taste, or are you looking at texture, aroma and appearance? Is the temperature important to you? Sometimes we need a mix of all flavours to feel truly satisfied. With flavours, we primarily look to balance sweet, salt, bitter, sour and umami, but I love working with textures too. Sweet, salty, crunchy and soft is a magical combination and one I believe to be most satisfying. Whenever I am explaining this to women at my events and workshops, I make my raw Key lime pie, which balances this combination and is sweet and salty. I'm yet to find a research paper to prove this so, for now, I go purely on the pleasure it gives me, and the feedback I've had from others.

Obviously eating intuitively isn't always going to be easy. Work commitments and time constraints mean that, occasionally, you aren't going to be able to eat exactly as you would like. You might need to eat something before taking a long trip, or eat a meal a friend has cooked for you, even though it wasn't really what you had in mind for that meal. That's okay. Learn to be flexible and enjoy eating – most importantly, guilt-free.

TASK: WHAT'S YOUR FLAVOUR?

Make a list of your favourite meals. Next to them, use the three categories or make up names that resonate more with you. When you're done, list them again, perhaps on something you can print off or see in your kitchen. Here you have a simple guide to eating intuitively. When you ask yourself how you want food to make you feel today, you've got your go-to guide.

REWRITING YOUR STORY: CONNECTING WITH THE FUTURE YOU

So how do you move forwards from here? What's the bigger picture for you, your body, your satisfaction, your intuitive life? Remember that it is your life and your decisions. Now that you have learnt what imprints and stories you've been carrying around like a ton of tins, you can recognise which need to be let go. These things we carry do not define us.

I want you to start thinking about what your version of success looks like. How do you feel after reading this book? How has it made you think about how you want to feel in your body and around food? This next exercise is something I learnt a while ago and it was an absolute game-changer for me. The journey of intuitive eating and living for me turned around when I took the time to invest in thinking about my future self. Instead of carrying around the old stories, I created a new one. The new me. Of course my physical body hadn't changed, but the way I approached life did.

VISUALISE YOUR FUTURE SELF

In my training as a life coach, I learnt a technique whereby you visualise your future self. It was so powerful for me in many ways. I saw her strength, her power, her wisdom. She wasn't afraid of her body. She was embodied. In the first meditation you speak with your future self and ask for her guidance. In the second meditation, you step into her life, allowing you to become her in feeling and spirit. You can use meditation one (see below) once or more if you feel like you need to reconnect with your future self and ask for guidance. Meditation two is for weekly use, enabling you to get closer to her each time.

Before you begin, have a think about how you imagine your future self. What does she do? What clothes does she wear? How does she satisfy herself? Where does she live? How does she move? How does she feel in her body? What does she eat?

Try to choose a time when you are already relaxed, so perhaps do some deep breathing or take a long bath beforehand. Let's begin . . .

MEDITATION ONE

Set some time aside to visualise your future self. Start by closing your eyes and taking three long, deep breaths. Relax into this moment, going deeper into a calm state with each exhale. Now, in your mind's eye, bring your awareness to your third-eye chakra, in between your brows. Imagine a bright white or golden light radiating from above you into this space and up into the crown of the head. With every inhale it brings in more light and takes away any darkness. With every exhale you feel lighter. Now imagine this bright white light radiating from the crown of the head down through the back of the body and into the earth from your feet. You may feel your feet tingle here. Now, as you inhale, bring that light back up through the front of your body and up through the crown of your head. Repeat this five times at your own pace, focusing on the breath as you go. Now, bring your attention to the room and imagine a magic carpet in front of you; walk towards it and feel the texture on your feet. Allow this magic carpet to take you to your favourite place in nature 20 years from now. Notice where in the world you are. Now use your senses; what can you see, hear, smell, touch and taste in the air? How do you feel here? In the distance you see your future self. Walk towards her and look her in the eye. Connect deeply. Ask her, 'What do I need to know? What steps do I need to take to get to you? How can I live my authentic self?' Now listen. Take in the surroundings, what you see and how you feel. Her answer may come in different ways. Ask any other questions you feel you need answers to. Give yourself time with her. Listen. When you are ready, look her deeply in the eye again and give her a hug, and thank her for her wisdom and guidance. Find your magic carpet and allow it to lift you up and bring you back into the room. Wiggle your fingers and toes here and take three long, deep breaths. When you are ready, slowly open your eyes, and come back into the physical world.

Want to listen to the meditations from this book? Download yours for free at www.rootedliving.co/intuitivelivingmeditations

When you're done, write down everything about this future self in your journal. Now answer the following questions:

- What do I need to get from where I am now, to my future self? List at least ten things.
- What questions do I need to ask my future self? (then go back to the visualisation and meet her again, asking these questions)
- How does my future self satisfy herself?
- How does my future self love herself?
- How does my future self feel in her body?
- What word does my future self embody?

Then think about a situation you are in that you want to change, or develop in to create more satisfaction in your life. Ask yourself: what would my future self do in this situation? Get to know your future self like a best friend or new lover. You want to know everything about her and more.

MEDITATION TWO

For the second meditation, use your magic carpet to take you to your favourite place as before. From here, imagine a door in front of you. There are ten steps down to the door. As you walk down each stair count from ten to one. You find yourself in a beautiful room. What does it look like? Now use your senses; what can you see, hear, smell, touch and taste in the air? How do you feel here? In front of you there is a screen. Here you see your future self – what is she doing? What life is she living, where and how? See her life on this screen and, after a few minutes, step into the screen and become her. Start living that life now. Embody that life now. How does that feel? Take time here to create this life. How do you feel in your body? How do you walk, talk, eat? When you're ready, slowly find the door that you came in through. There are now ten steps up to it so count from one to ten as you walk up slowly. As you come out of the door you find your magic carpet. Allow it to lift you up and bring you back into the room. Wiggle your fingers and toes here and take three long, deep breaths. When you are ready, slowly open your eyes, and come back into the physical world.

Do this visualisation weekly, and let your future self guide you. Step into this life with daily experiences. Check in with her each morning – what would she wear? What would she eat? How would she step into the situation you're in? You are the author of your story. You are ready to live intuitively. Welcome to the movement.

TRANSITIONS: IMPLEMENTING CHANGE

Not all positive changes feel positive in the beginning. Nothing is fixed and transformation happens all the time. From the cells in our body, our consciousness and the choices we make in life, we are constantly evolving. There is so much emphasis on the New Year, or the freshness of September as we relive the feeling of going back to school, but every moment in time is an opportunity for growth and change. How do we implement changes throughout the way we live intuitively? What happens if and when we feel overwhelmed with this new intuitive life? Trust the process; your intuition is always on your side. In this section I'll be supporting you to notice and trust transitions, big and small, and show you that you can be both achieving and transitioning, while also being a work-in-progress.

You may have earmarked many pages within this book that resonated with you. There may be passages you feel you need to explore further or tools that you are still resisting. This all comes in time. Remember, it's the small transitions that have the biggest impact. Tweaks each day, week and month as opposed to one huge overhaul that is yet another opportunity to feel overwhelmed or lost. What can you do today? Know that there is no rush. In reading this book you have started a beautiful journey, back to yourself. Change can be hard, so below I've listed my top tips to keeping transitions simpler and a little less stressful:

1. If getting from A to B feels overwhelming, break up large-scale changes to smaller ones; make them more manageable.
2. Link changes into a routine or ritual, to allow a smooth transition. For example, if you know that meditating enhances your ability to eat intuitively, you can try doing it on your daily commute so it doesn't take up additional time in the day.
3. Accept change, don't resist it. Repeat after me: I accept . . . .
4. Don't predict the future. Fear will try to get in the way by creating stories in your head about how the outcome might play out. While we can anticipate certain elements that a change might bring, it is impossible to know everything that will happen in advance.
5. Be prepared for surprises, and the winds of change won't easily knock you over.

TASK: I AM, BUT STILL

Who you are reading this right now is different from the person you were this morning. You are different from who you will be tomorrow, next month or next year. While change is important, honouring our many facets allows us to really sit within the feminine. Give yourself permission to be strong. Give yourself permission to be vulnerable. Explore this via this task in your journal.

I am ...., but still ....

For example:

I am growing, but still learning.
I am strong, but still sensitive.
I am authentic, but still exploring new parts of myself.
I am enough, but still growing.
I am confident, but still vulnerable.

CASE STUDY: CLAIRE

You are allowed to underachieve. You are allowed to strive to be a masterpiece but also to be a work-in-progress, in the process. This was so true for a client I worked with. Claire strived for her idea of perfection in everything she did. Everything she did was about how she would be seen, but in doing so she was far away from the person she really was. Claire came to me because she had issues with food and felt that constantly counting calories was causing her to feel overwhelmed. She also had high expectations of herself – in everything from exercise to her career, which was causing her anxiety and also affecting her relationship. Together, we started to look at the causes of her high expectations, most of which came from her upbringing where she tried to compete with her brother who the family thought of as more intelligent. She struggled to be like him and this had stuck. We worked on what made Claire unique and what her personal qualities were; her abilities, strengths and passions. I then asked Claire to tell me where she was still progressing, what she felt she lacked in life and why she thought this should be deemed as failure. In doing so, Claire realised that this progress was where she was doing her greatest work. Through the cracks she saw the light. She learnt that by lumbering herself with high expectations all the time, she was setting herself up to fail. One by one we looked at where she could let go of things in her life that weren't serving her. Meal by meal, she stopped counting calories and, instead, ate for nourishment, guided by what her body needed. She started exercising based on how she wanted to feel, and not because she felt it would make her stay slim. She started to be honest about her feelings, rather than hide them away through fear of being judged. She started showing people the real her.

Nothing is definitive. There is no one perfect route to living intuitively, just like there is no one perfect handbook for life. Trust that there is learning in everything and that to be vulnerable and honest about your feelings will be your greatest gift. We can be both hard on the outside and soft on the inside. In fact, this I believe is the most magical combination.

MANIFESTING MAGIC

Now it's time to talk about creating more of the good stuff. You're on the road to satisfaction and you're feeling inspired (I hope) by the previous five chapters of this book. In this section we look at ways to keep on keeping on with the high vibes both for body-love and intuitive living. Here are some of my favourite tools for manifesting magic.

Manifesting is intentionally creating what you want. Everyone has the ability to manifest anything they desire – wealth, optimum health, love, houses, cars, peace of mind – it's just that we're not taught this growing up. The power to manifest lies within you. You just have to learn how to use it. The idea behind manifesting is that whatever you think about, you are manifesting into your life. Similar to what we've explored with toxic self-talk, if you're telling yourself you're not worthy, think about the negativity you'll be absorbing. If you tell yourself you're confident and successful, how could that play out? Much better! If you are constantly thinking about what you don't want to happen, that is exactly what you are manifesting. But by learning to use manifesting, you are instantly beginning to change your thoughts and your beliefs. You can remain focused on what you want to happen, allowing your greatest desires to manifest.

Everything happening in your life is a reflection of what is happening inside of you. Whatever you focus on will take shape and manifest into your daily life, in the same way as how you talk to yourself. You talk kinder, you feel better. The topic of manifesting is a far greater subject, and a whole other book, but after the work you've done up to this point, it's important to recognise your ability to create how you want to feel and be in this world. These tips are considered spiritual bypassing so they certainly won't shift you into being a deep manifester or creator, but they will open you up to the possibility of feeling the best you can each day and living a transformative intuitive life.

EXPANDING

Expanding supports you by calling in your desires and brings in an abundance of support to help you own your journey into intuitive living and manifesting magic. Change can be challenging. It's unfamiliar and not always an easy process but, by expanding, you create the support network. For example, in your vision for yourself in the future, you feel vibrant and healthy. You are confident in your body. You have a new job in the arts where you feel successful and worthy. Fear might try to get in the way of this with feelings of frustration or doubt that rise up to the surface faster than the speed of light. This is totally normal and a way in which the universe tests you. You overcome the fear by expanding. How can you step into this new you and this new job? How do you need to start thinking and feeling? Bring it back to the vision of your future self. What would she do? But on a more practical level, who do you need to surround yourself with in order to reach this goal? You must go and expand your subconscious structure of belief through completely immersing yourself in your vision. Can you start a class or go to a workshop that will surround you with like-minded people? Can you buddy up with a friend who you know is going through similar transitions and be each other's support network? Maybe you need to embrace a life coach to support you. Expanding is not only shaping how we think but putting the action into place. Start with the willingness to transform, and expand into it.

THOUGHTS NEED FEELING

The fastest way to create more of the good stuff in your life is to actively put emphasis on feeling good. When it comes to intuitive living, we can think about what we want until the cows come home, but the secret is in the feeling. For example, it's all very well saying, 'I want to be more confident', but how will it feel to be confident, and can you embody that feeling right now? Let's put this into perspective. Think about a day when you wake up in a great mood, you get a seat on the train or bus to work and then, when you get to work, someone has left you a coffee on your desk and your boss calls you in to say you won the new account you'd been working on. Your day is good because you set the tone for it. It's as simple as that.

The law of attraction always has your back by giving you more situations that match the high vibe that you're putting out there. That's exactly how it works. When you're *feeling* happy and full of high vibes, you're creating the conditions that dictate that, no matter what happens that day, it's going to be a good 'un. Then, in turn, the universe shows up and helps you to make that happen. Now, I'm not saying every day is going to be golden, but think about what vibrations you are sending out. Choose them carefully!

Why not try it out for yourself? Create a morning ritual that you know puts you in a high-vibe state. Write your gratitude journal focusing on things that are really supporting you in life and bring the feeling into why it's good. Feeling good is a choice, so keep coming back to it.

VISION BOARDS

Any theory about visualising your goals will tell you that in order to attract what you truly want, you must see it, you must feel it, and you must embody it. Having only one of these lessens the effectiveness. I love creating vision boards as a way to get creative with my life goals and to be reminded visually of them each day. The big secret to creating a vision board that works is simple: your vision board should focus on how you want to feel, not just on things that you want. Don't get me wrong, it's great to include the material stuff too; however, the more your board focuses on how you want to feel, the more it will come to life. In other words, pictures alone aren't going to move the needle. You've got to understand the feeling behind the image.

Step 1: Make a list of the areas of your life that are most important to you. Maybe you've been daydreaming about the perfect partner or a bigger salary or a far-flung holiday destination that seems totally unattainable. Light a candle and take some space for you to tune in and clarify what you really want, including all of the juicy details. You may want to start with a stream of consciousness, writing everything down just to get your initial thoughts out, and then identify the stuff that really lights you up. This might sound cheesy but really it's not, it's called focus. And when was the last time you really identified and focused on what you wanted?

Step 2: What should you put on your vision board? There are no hard-and-fast rules here so add anything that inspires and motivates you. The purpose of your vision board is to bring everything on it to life. First, think about what your goals are in the different areas of your life (you can use the satisfaction planner from the previous chapter as a guide) and then find an image that embodies the feeling associated with it. For example, how will you feel when you meet this new partner, or when the higher salary lands in your bank account? You don't have to cover each area exactly the same, just take a mental inventory of what you want each of those areas to look like and write them down. I find hand-writing specific goals instead of typing them – such as money goals – more powerful. There's always something energetically special about actually writing your goals by hand – visual representation of them for your board. Don't overthink it, just go with your gut and have fun. If you want to retrain as a nutrition coach, select photos of inspiring food. If you want to be a beauty expert, use some natural beauty images. Or if you want to call in an abundance, of success, perhaps include photos of entrepreneurial or successful women who you aspire to be like. For a BFF-style pep talk, add motivational words that represent how you want to feel. The world is your oyster.

Step 3: Connect with your vision board. Now that you've tapped into what you really want, give yourself time to look at it. To get the full benefit from your vision board, it's important for you to place it somewhere you can see it every day. I recommend you take a few minutes to look over your vision board at least once or twice a day. I like to review my vision board right before I do a guided visualisation, so my goals are at the forefront of my mind as I train it to attract what I truly want into my life. I also like to review it every night before I go to sleep, in order to prompt my subconscious mind to come up with new ideas while I'm sleeping on how to achieve my goals. That way, I wake up in the morning bursting with motivation to succeed – and am far more likely to notice and act on opportunities that will bring me closer to my goals.

You can recreate your board whenever it feels right. I tend to prune mine as I go through the year, but always really check in with it in January and at the six-month mark, in July, when my real new year starts – my birthday! The more excited you get about what you want to create, the more likely it is you'll attract it into your life.

Some additional ways to connect with your completed vision board:

- Look at your vision board often – daily is best.
- Tap into how it makes you feel – satisfied and inspired by your life.
- Read your daily affirmations and inspirational words out loud. Feel their power.
- See and feel yourself living in your goals and visions.
- Feel yourself in the future you have designed in your vision board.
- Believe it is already yours.
- Be grateful for the good that is already present in your life.
- Celebrate any goals you have already achieved.
- Acknowledge the changes you have seen and felt.

STAYING ON THE RAILS (FAQS)

This section is a compilation of the most common questions I get asked about body-love and intuitive eating and living. From clients I've worked with one to one, to the hundreds of women on my programmes, there are always similar questions that come up, so view this as your one-stop shop for staying on the rails.

Can I eat intuitively all the time? What happens when I'm on holiday or the choice is out of my control?

No, it's inevitable that life will get in the way sometimes. You may eat something that doesn't feel right or eat past the point of fullness because a) life happens and b) sometimes it's fun. But what we don't want here is for you to feel like a failure, putting you right back into the diet cycle of shame followed by restriction followed by overeating followed by shame again. Take it on the chin, eat, don't give yourself the guilt trip and move on the next day. Intuitive eating allows flexibility, so take it with hands wide open.

What happens if I go off the rails and use food to make me feel good or eat emotionally?

If you do find yourself in the middle of a binge, just take note of the situation and try allowing yourself to fully enjoy it, rather than fighting it. Sometimes we all just need a piece of cake. Sit down and savour every bite. The more focused you are on how good it feels to eat, the harder it will be to eat to the point of pain. When we eat emotionally, it is usually an attempt by our bodies to experience pleasure. Allow yourself to explore other ways to experience feeling good, aside from eating.

I overeat due to a fear of scarcity. What can I do to support myself in staying on the intuitive eating journey?

Always carry food with you so that you never feel deprived. Emotional eating can be your body's reaction to feeling deprived, so create new ways to nourish yourself. Stock your fridge with delicious, healthy foods, pack your calendar with exciting things to do, and be disciplined about setting aside time for yourself to relax.

Intuitive eating is all about putting weight loss on the back burner but how can I be sure I get there and know I'm not secretly trying to lose the weight?

Beware of pseudo-dieting. This is when you think you're on top of your intuitive eating but secretly you are finding it hard to shake the mentality. For example, you might be cutting out certain macronutrients after 6pm even though you are hungry and intuitively feel like you need them. Or you might find yourself cutting back on food before an event or party. I realise it can be difficult to find the loopholes in your own eating patterns and behaviour if you aren't completely sure what to be looking out for. This is where I would take to your journal and write down your emotions around foods. Can you notice something around the way you eat and how it makes you feel? What do you think when eating certain foods? If in doubt, get support from a professional.

How do you show yourself unconditional love when you really do not love that extra tyre around your belly or the excess fat on your thighs?

I think it's important to note that unconditional love for your body is a journey back to the self. Self-love, in caring for you as a whole, is one thing, but you may not always love your body. Start the process by finding acceptance of your body, its uses and the support it gives you in life. Your body chose you. Talk to your body; perhaps the bits you like first and then move on to the bits you dislike. Can you list some reasons why – even though you feel it isn't worthy (which of course it is) – your body deserves to be loved? Sometimes you have to see it to believe it.

How do you make sure you listen to your intuition rather than the naughty negative voice? I can very often hear it but I just don't listen to it.

Tap into why you are resisting it. Is your intuition telling you something you know may open a can of worms? Self-development isn't always easy and, when we are choosing to live with the toxic self-talk over our intuition, it's usually because we are keeping ourselves safe.

If I give myself full permission to eat everything I'm so afraid I'll just eat junk food and never stop eating. How can I make sure this won't happen?

I completely understand this concern. Let's imagine you allow yourself a pizza for dinner when you usually wouldn't. At first the thought may excite you, but how do you think you'll feel if you allowed yourself pizza for dinner every single night of the week? Eventually you'll get to food habituation, which is when the novelty and reward stimulated by a certain food wears off. It doesn't seem so desirable anymore. Plus, I might be wrong but intuitively, I don't think your body would feel great eating pizza every single night. You may start to feel sluggish. Yes, intuitive eating gives you permission to eat what you want but it also encourages you to tune in to hunger and fullness, so, long term, you stop overeating. I guarantee that constantly eating foods that aren't nutrient-dense for a long period of time will not make you feel good, but you will only learn this with direct experience and trust.

How long will it take me to become an intuitive eater?

I can't give you an answer to this one because each person has their own timeline. It really depends on your dieting history, the root causes and how dysfunctional your relationship with food is. The more disordered your eating is and the longer you have been in a diet mentality, the longer it may take you. Equally, I've seen people transforming in a matter of weeks. Some people can learn to be intuitive eaters in just a few months, others need years (such as those with eating disorders). The good news is that there is light at the end of what can often be a very dark tunnel. You will eventually get to a place of peace with food.

DO YOU (THE MANIFESTO)

I have an incredible girl gang; two women, Sara and Katie, who truly understand me, support me and inspire me. Katie's mum always says to her, 'You do you' and we say it all the time in jest. But there is such truth in these three simple words. I started this book explaining how you are the centre of your universe. I end this book encouraging you to do YOU. Intuitive Living is the new movement. No more clean eating, chasing gurus and finding wisdom from outside of yourself. The wisdom is within you.

Everyone's spiritual path is *their* path and we can only trust in nature's course. There will always be someone who might judge, try to trip you up, compare against you or try to dim your light. But by creating and expanding your own inner light on an ongoing basis, you make sure to tend to your own energy field and your own abundant, intuitive life. We are all connected by the same source energy. We all are source energy. In the world of intuition and soul there is no I, but we. We work together with the flows and rhythms of nature. When you open your heart wide enough to desire the same level of consciousness for others as you want for yourself, you put a vibrant energy into motion. This is intuitive living.

In transforming your life to live intuitively, you reconnect to areas you've been hiding from, and break free from lies you've been living and from blocks that have kept you stuck. As your life transforms, so does your relationship with food and your body. You rid yourself of old beliefs and stop playing small and, instead, start showing up for yourself in a big way. I know this because I've seen it. You can feel empowered when you empower other people. I used to say that I help to empower women, but now I know I don't empower them – I see their power and help them to see it too. I hope that, in reading this book, you feel empowered; feel brave enough to shine your light wide and far. To all of you divine females, today and every day – be kind, to yourself and to others. Don't play small. Honour yourself. Trust yourself. Trust that you can have it all. Show the world that you won't settle for less. Be YOU.

Here is MY Intuitive Living Manifesto for YOU:

- I agree, from this day forward, to fully engage in life on earth.
- I will inhabit the vehicle that chose me – my body – and keep it loved and safe from this day forward.
- I will nourish this body with nutritious food, pleasure, kindness and compassion.
- I will speak to this body only with kindness and acceptance.
- I acknowledge that my body will change from infancy to old age and I will accept it in this process.
- I recognise that my body will call for different foods as the days, seasons and years progress. I understand that there is no one perfect diet.
- I honour that, as a woman, I have a special relationship with eating and nourishment.
- I will cultivate my own unique sense of beauty.
- I will engage in self-discovery and self-knowledge.
- I recognise that, at its deepest level, eating is an affirmation of life.
- I will honour when I need to say no, and trust to say yes to overcome irrational fears.
- I will honour my inner child and listen to her needs.
- I will surround myself with positive people who love and encourage me.
- I will dream big.
- I will trust myself and my intuition.
- I will concentrate on my story and my journey.
- I will love my story and my journey.
- I will be patient with myself.

- I will honour the stillness I need to rest.
- I will expand and explore always.

'Don't be satisfied with stories, how things have gone with others. Unfold your own myth.' Rumi

References

WEEK 1: SELF-LOVE IS TRUE LOVE

1. Fredrickson, B. L. et al. 'Open Hearts Build Lives: Positive Emotions, Induced Through Loving-Kindness Meditation, Build Consequential Personal Resources', *Journal of Personality and Social Psychology* (Nov 2008) 95(5): 1045–62.
2. Robles, T. F. and Carroll, J. E. 'Restorative biological processes and health', *Social and Personality Psychology Compass* (Aug 2011) 5(8): 518–37.
3. Homan, K. J. and Tylka, T. L. 'Development and exploration of the gratitude model of body appreciation in women', *Body Image* (June 2018) 25: 14–22.
4. Theodoridou, A. et al. 'Oxytocin and social perception: Oxytocin increases perceived facial trustworthiness and attractiveness', *Hormones and Behavior* (June 2009) 56(1): 128–32.
5. Zak, P. J., Stanton, A. A. and Ahmadi, S. 'Oxytocin Increases Generosity in Humans', *PLoS ONE* (Nov 2007) 2(11): 1128–371.

WEEK 2: YOU ARE WHAT YOU THINK

1. Salk, R. H. and Engeln-Maddox, R. 'If You're Fat, Then I'm Humongous!', *Psychology of Women Quarterly* (March 2011) 35(1): 18–28.
2. Stewart-Brown, S. 'Emotional wellbeing and its relation to health', *BMJ* (Dec 1998) 317(7173): 1608–09.

3. Kuss, D. J. and Griffiths, M. D. 'Online Social Networking and Addiction – A Review of the Psychological Literature', *International Journal of Environmental Research and Public Health* (Sep 2011) 8(9): 3528–52.

WEEK 3: LISTEN TO YOUR BODY – UNDERSTANDING INTUITION

1. Gur, R. C. and Gur, R. E. 'Complementarity of Sex Differences in Brain and Behaviour: From Laterality to Multi-Modal Neuroimaging', *Journal of Neuroscience Research* (Jan 2017) 95(1–2): 189–99.
2. Colom, R. et al. 'Hippocampal structure and human cognition', *Intelligence* (March 2013) 41(2): 129–40.

WEEK 4: FEED YOUR SOUL

1. Redman, L. M. and Ravussin, E. 'Caloric Restriction in Humans: Impact on Physiological, Psychological, and Behavioral Outcomes', *Antioxidants and Redox Signaling* (Jan 2015) 14(2): 275–87.
2. MacLean, P. S. et al. 'Biology's Response to Dieting: The impetus for weight regain', *American Journal of Physiology-Regulatory, Integrative and Comparative Physiology* (Sep 2011) 301(3): 581–600.
3. Kiortsis, D. N., Durack, I. and Turpin, G. 'Effects of a low-calorie diet on resting metabolic rate and serum tri-iodothyronine levels in obese children', *European Journal of Pediatrics* (Jun 1999) 158(6): 446–50.
4. Kasper, J. M., Johnson, S. B. and Hommel, J. D. 'Fat Preference: A novel model of eating behavior in rats', *Journal of Visualized Experiments* (June 2014) (88): e51575.
5. Fuhrman, J. et al. 'Changing perceptions of hunger on a high nutrient density diet', *Nutrition Journal* (Nov 2010) 9: 51.
6. intuitiveeating.com/resources/articles
7. Pietiläinen, K. H. et al. 'Does dieting make you fat? A twin study',

International Journal of Obesity (March 2012) 36(3): 456–64.

8. beateatingdisorders.org.uk/types/emotional-overeating
9. Taheri, S. et al. 'Short sleep duration is associated with reduced leptin, elevated ghrelin, and increased body mass index', *PLoS Medicine* (Dec 2004) 1(3): e62.
10. Daubenmier, J. et al. 'Mindfulness Intervention for Stress Eating to Reduce Cortisol and Abdominal Fat among Overweight and Obese Women', *Journal of Obesity* (2011) 651936.

WEEK 5: FINDING SATISFACTION

1. Saris, W. E. et al. *A comparative study of satisfaction with life in Europe*, (Budapest, 1996), pp. 11–48.
2. Ghent, A. 'The happiness effect', *Bulletin World Health Organization* (Apr 2011) 89(4): 246–7.
3. Ibid.
4. Kimura, D. 'Work and Life Balance: "If We Are Not Happy Both in Work and out of Work, We Cannot Provide Happiness to Others"', *Frontiers in Pediatrics* (Feb 2016) 4:9.
5. Lyubomirsky, S., Sheldon, K. M. and Schkade, D. 'Pursuing Happiness: The Architecture of Sustainable Change', *Review of General Psychology* (2005) 9(2): 111–31.
6. Faith, M. S. et al. 'Parent–child feeding strategies and their relationships to child eating and weight status', *Obesity Research* (Nov 2004) 12(11): 1711–22.
7. Ibid.
8. Chu, Y. L. et al. 'Involvement in home meal preparation is associated with food preference and self-efficacy among Canadian children', *Public Health Nutrition* (Jan 2013) 16(1): 108–12
9. Avena, N. M., Murray, S. and Gold, M. S. 'Comparing the effects of food restriction and overeating on brain reward systems', *Experimental Gerontology* (Oct 2013) 48(10): 1062–7.

10. Keast, R. S. J and Costanzo, A. 'Is fat the sixth taste primary? Evidence and implications', *Flavour* (2015) 4(5): 1–7.

11. Majeed, H. and Moore, G. W. K. 'Impact of Multidecadal Climate Variability on United Kingdom Rickets Rates', *Scientific Reports* (Nov 2017) 7(1).

12. Volkow, N. D., Wang, G. J. and Baler, R. D. 'Reward, dopamine and the control of food intake: implications for obesity', *Trends in Cognitive Science* (Jan 2011) 15(1): 37–46.

13. Oldham-Cooper, R. E. et al. 'Playing a computer game during lunch affects fullness, memory for lunch, and later snack intake', *American Journal of Clinical Nutrition* (Feb 2011) 93(2): 308–13.

14. Harvard Study of Adult Development: adultdevelopmentstudy.org

Acknowledgements

To my girl gang, Katie and Sara (the GG unit), Emily and Kate and all of the women who I have met, laughed with and loved throughout the years. Without your love and support, I am nothing.

To my mother, who is the strongest, most badass, brave babe there is. You did good, Mum. I love and respect you with my whole heart.

To my team, Olivia Morris and Ru Merritt at Orion, my agent Valeria Huerta and her assistant Olivia Percival, my amazing assistant and friend, Abi Lough and my designer and illustrator, Cris Jones. Thank you all for your support.

To my clients. You have all inspired me with your wisdom, courage, strength and feminine force. You have trusted me to hold you and support you and I am forever grateful. Go and show the world who you are and continue to inspire others to do the same.

To my life partner and rock, Tom. Meeting you and sharing the world together has shaped me in all areas of life. Thank you for always challenging me, believing in me and being by my side in this wild ride called life. You are my world.

To women everywhere. Know that you have innate wisdom and power within you, that life is always ready for you to show up to your authentic self. Self-love is your foundation. Don't ever forget yourself and your needs.

Finally to my daughter, Romilly. In giving you life, you have given me life in ways I didn't believe possible. Expand and explore always my darling and don't ever let anyone dim your light. I love you to the moon and back.

About the Author

Pandora Paloma is an Intuitive Living Coach, specialising in Intuitive Eating and Living. She is an author, speaker and teacher, spreading the movement of Intuitive Living worldwide.

Drawing on her own battle with food and body image, along with her unique training as a Nutritionist, Intuitive Eating specialist, Life Coach, Yoga teacher and Meditation guide, it is her mission to be a voice for women. A voice that stands up and says, 'You are so much more than your body and your weight does not define you.' Her work inspires women to rebel against society's beauty standards and instead feel safe, supported and empowered in the skin they are in. She is a big believer in listening to your body and feeding your soul – believing that optimum health starts with loving yourself, your body and your mind.

She has shared her message with residencies and speaking events with Soho House Group, Spotify, Nicholas Kirkwood, Bare Minerals, Lulu Lemon, Stylist LIVE and Topshop. Pandora regularly provides advice and comment for the UK's leading magazines including *Stylist*, *Grazia*, *Get the Gloss*, *Byrdie UK* and *Women's Health*, and has been featured in *Elle*, *Psychologies*, *Refinery 29*, *Harper's Bazaar* and *Evening Standard*.

When Pandora isn't spreading self-love, the power of intuition and female empowerment, she is found walking on beaches in Kent, dancing to techno and cooking and eating (intuitively of course).